KNEE SURGERY

The Essential Guide to Total Knee Recovery

KNEE SURGERY

The Essential Guide to Total Knee Recovery

Daniel Fulham O'Neill, M.D., Ed.D.

ST. MARTIN'S GRIFFIN ❧ NEW YORK

www.stmartins.com

Book design by / Maura Fadden Rosenthal

Photography copyright © 2008 by Michael Patrick O'Neill,
www.ONeillImages.com
Illustrations copyright © 2008 by Keith Morrissey and
Amanda Condict

Library of Congress Cataloging-in-Publication Data

O'Neill, Daniel Fulham.
    Knee surgery : the essential guide to total knee recovery /
Daniel Fulham O'Neill.
        p. cm.
    ISBN-13: 978-0-312-36293-5
    ISBN-10: 0-312-36293-5
    1. Knee—Surgery—Popular works.   I. Title.
    RD561.O54 2008
    617.5'82059—dc22

                                    2008025262

10 9 8 7 6 5 4 3

For my three Patricias

CONTENTS

ILLUSTRATIONS

ACKNOWLEDGMENTS

DOCTORS SHOULD NEVER use the word *I*, because the voices of teachers, colleagues, and especially patients are constantly channeling through our minds. As a doctor, then, it is important to say that these are the people who actually wrote this book.

I have been lucky to work with an inspiring group over the years:

From the old New Hampshire Knee Center: Debbie Hoefs, Jim Nolan, Janine Mauche-Dumond, Lynne Bates, Bill Knowles, Katie Grant, and Kara LaMarche.

The latest Alpine Clinic players: Mia Simone, Gretchen Wilkie, and lifers Marie Simpson and Mark "Cabbie" McGlone.

For their help with the manuscript: Patrick Dimick; D'Anne Bodman, a great poet and friend; and Keith Morrissey, my illustrator.

For their support from the beginning (literally): the O'Neill family, especially my photographer, Michael Patrick O'Neill; cousin Janis Harrington; and CuChulain.

For bringing this project to fruition: the unstoppable Daryl Browne; my agent, Fran Collin; my editor, Regina Scarpa; and my copy editor, Cynthia Merman.

Finally, thank you to just a few of my mentors: Jim Cardon, Jake Stearns, Stu Cherney, Bruce Meinhard, Stan James, Len Zaichkowsky, K. Donald Shelbourne, and the incomparable Hilton Weiss.

KNEE SURGERY

The Essential Guide to Total Knee Recovery

INTRODUCTION

WHEN I BEGAN my medical practice in orthopedics, there was no concise source for reliable patient information regarding knee surgery, much less one describing all the little things that can help people before and after the operation. To address this, I wrote handouts for my patients to reinforce what we had discussed in the office. When my handout grew to 160 pages and I began to get calls from colleagues and folks all over the country looking for a copy, I decided it was time to write a proper book. One nice thing about knees is that they are almost all rehabilitated in the same way. So here it is: information you can actually use to get your knee working the way you want it to—or maybe even better!

According to the American Academy of Orthopaedic Surgeons, four hundred thousand people in the United States will have total knee replacement (TKR) surgery this year. Another one hundred thousand will have their ACL (anterior cruciate ligament) reconstructed, and millions will have "simple" knee arthroscopies for a variety of cartilage tears, scar tissue, minor arthritis, etc. (Although as your surgeon will tell you, there is nothing "simple" about it.) Good operations are being performed by good surgeons, but patients are not always given the guidance they need to get better quickly, reliably, and yes, inexpensively. In other words, someone you know will be having knee surgery soon and needs to read this book!

Besides the physical stress, surgery is a strain psychologically. Thus, effective healing needs to take place on both fronts. Unfortunately, being a surgeon does not train you to understand the mental side of injury and recovery. To remedy this, a few years ago I went back to school for a degree in sports psychology to better understand the mind-body connection. We all see this connection daily, but because of its ethereal nature, very few doctors address it consistently with their patients. Ultimately, I want you to approach your knee surgery like Lance Armstrong before riding the Alps: as strong as possible both physically and mentally!

Knee Surgery: The Essential Guide to Total Knee Recovery is the first book written by an expert in the field that combines both physical and mental rehabilitation after common knee surgeries in a simple, easy-to-follow program. Busy doctors, therapists, and athletic trainers have limited time to spend on an individual's physical *and* mental rehabilitation—*yet these are keys to your full recovery.* Working together with your medical team and this book, you can maximize the efficiency of your rehabilitation program. Healing from common knee operations is relatively straightforward—if you are empowered and properly coached.

This book is just such a coach, answering your questions and providing the daily tools you will need for a complete physical and mental return to your life after knee injury or surgery. I promise you that on every page of this book you will find useful information to make your knee better in the short and long terms. When used properly, this book will save you loads of time and buckets of money, and, perhaps most important, save you from unnecessary pain.

As a teenager with little cash and even less knowledge of car engines, I was lucky to stumble upon a book called *How to Keep Your Volkswagen Alive: A Manual of Step-by-Step Procedures for the Complete Idiot.* This book not only helped me to keep my '68 Beetle going, it also made me realize that complex topics could be explained succinctly and entertainingly. I have refined my rehab program over the years on this model to give you only the information and activities you need to get back to your life—I hope with a smile on your face!

The program is divided into three "prongs" consisting of *exercises*, including range-of-motion (ROM) stretches; *movement patterns/sports* to keep your muscle memory alive for your return to normal activities; and *aerobic training* to help you regain your endurance and stamina. Each prong is divided into multiple levels of increasing difficulty until your

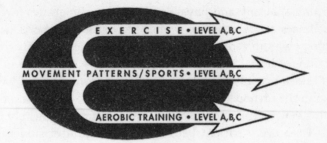

Three-pronged attack

knee is ready for everything that life throws at it—including the New England winters that my patients have to endure. The three-pronged attack may look complicated at first, but trust me: I have eliminated all of the fat and given you only what you need to get off the couch and back to action.

Many people look at knee surgery, especially arthroscopic knee surgery, as "keyhole" or "minor" surgery and expect to be back full-time, full-speed within days. The expectation is similar for ligament surgery (which, like arthroscopic knee surgery, is also often done as an outpatient procedure) and is not much different for the mother of all knee surgeries, the total knee replacement. People believe that they can pop into the hospital one morning, go home that afternoon, and in the evening get on with life. In my clinic I do my best to dispel this myth. Our philosophy is simple: THERE IS NO SUCH THING AS MINOR SURGERY IF IT'S YOUR BODY! Knowing what you are getting into ahead of time will allow things to go smoother, will be less stressful, and will ultimately lead to a better result. It does, however, take some work on your part.

Unlike professional athletes, most people who come to a physician's office have continued playing and working on their less-than-healthy knees for many months. Pain prevents normal knee function, causing the muscles to grow weak—along with the spirit. I wrote this book to be a thinking person's guide to knee rehabilitation, acknowledging that there are also mental aspects of injury and recovery. After years of learning anatomy and physiology, doctors sometimes forget that knees are attached to a brain. My study of sports psychology was an attempt to understand and exploit this connection for better and faster healing.

Besides my interest in the mind-body connection, I have been in the orthopedic trenches taking care of knees for more than twenty years. My patients' care is directed entirely by me—I see every patient before, during, and after surgery. I also keep a relatively low volume of patients so that I can maintain this hands-on approach. I know how long it takes for a forty-five-year-old knee with a torn cartilage to get better after surgery. I appreciate the vast difference between a professional athlete recovering from ACL reconstruction versus a professional mother with a full-time job and two kids. I have seen the ultimate struggle to regain motion after a total knee replacement in a knee that has not moved without pain for ten years. It is my sincere hope that what I have witnessed, learned, and now set down on paper will be of great help not only for patients but also for concerned medical practitioners of every stripe looking for improved results with their knee patients.

PART ONE

JOURNEY INTO SURGERY

THE ROAD TO KNEE SURGERY

The Anatomy and Pathology
You Need to Know Before
Starting Your Journey

WHETHER WE ARE making our way across an icy parking lot, stepping into a canoe, or just getting out of bed, all of us perform athletic maneuvers daily. When a knee injury becomes part of the equation, the way you get better is no different from the way Tiger Woods recovers. The activity level you return to might be different, but the road traveled is the same.

The knee is a strong, hardworking joint. It helps us walk, get in and out of cars, do yoga, play football, ride horses, etc. Every day we depend on our knees for literally thousands of movements—some that we perform intentionally and others we don't even think about. In spite of their strength, knees tend to get hurt. Whether from arthritis, athletics, or overuse, almost everyone will have knee pain at some point in his or her life. To complicate matters, the knee has a number of structures that simply do not heal after they are injured. This translates into lots of knees ending up on the operating table. If a knee operation is in your future, you are definitely not alone.

Whether your surgery is for an injury to the cartilage, ligament, tendon, or bone, the goal after the operation (post-op) is to get the knee joint moving fully and for your muscles to regain their functional qualities: balance, flexibility, coordination, strength, speed, and quickness. This is called rehabilitation, or rehab for short. An important part of rehab is having the right mental attitude. As you read the chapters that follow, you will learn concrete, practical steps for your physical and mental rehab that apply to the vast majority of knee injuries and surgeries. The care and feeding of all knees are alike, only the time lines for recovery vary.

Having knee surgery is a big deal and it's okay to be frustrated, angry, even scared. It is okay for *now*—not forever. Having any kind of physical problem can leave even the toughest person feeling vulnerable and mortal. The good news is that in the twenty-first century, medical technology can make almost any knee useful for most jobs and many sports. But let's not sugarcoat this: Recovery from knee surgery takes work. It's not like brain surgery where you either get better or you don't. Knee rehab involves a physical and mental process which, when performed properly and diligently, helps ensure a good, functional outcome. Another great thing about recovery from knee surgery is you get back more than what you put into it. Each stretch, each exercise, each movement pattern not only improves your knee but also works your back, your hips, your balance, and more. Getting into the habit of caring for your knee translates into caring for total fitness. Thus, with the right attitude, a good doctor, and this book, you will soon be speeding toward a healthier you!

ANATOMY AND PATHOLOGY
OF THE KNEE

Before I get started talking about surgery, it will be helpful to develop a working knowledge of the knee's parts and functions. This will help you communicate with your doctor and therapist. As a bonus, this section will also prepare you for future episodes of *Jeopardy!*

Anatomy

Orthopedic surgeons, physical therapists, athletic trainers, and other sports medicine professionals spend their lives caring for the *musculoskeletal system*. This system consists of *muscles*, which provide movement, and *bones*, which form your body's internal frame. Muscles consist of multiple fibers that get larger and more efficient with exercise. There are more than four hundred muscles in the body, connecting more than two hundred bones. The muscles attach themselves to the bones via *tendons*.

Ligaments are tough fibrous tissues that connect bones to other bones. Ligaments can be thought of as similar to ropes because they have no ability to change their length. Due to this ropelike quality, we refer to ligaments as "static stabilizers." Conversely, muscles and tendons shorten and lengthen with motion and thus are called "dynamic stabilizers." Luckily, many ligament tears heal naturally on their own with time and activity modification. The medial collateral ligament of the knee is one such ligament (discussed later in this chapter).

Despite reasonable care, certain ligaments do not repair themselves. These include the anterior cruciate ligament (ACL) (connecting the femur to the tibia) and the capsular ligaments in the shoulder (dislocated shoulder). A rehabilitation program for an ACL tear or a dislocated shoulder will attempt to strengthen the muscles and tendons around the joint, but unless these ligaments are repaired surgically, the joint will always be vulnerable.

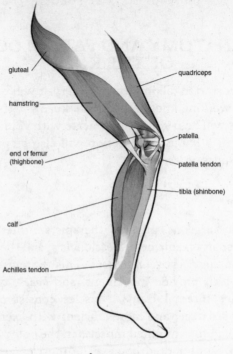

Leg anatomy

A *joint* is where two bones come together. At joints that have significant motion, the bone ends are covered with a smooth layer called *articular* or *surface cartilage*. In some joints, including the knee, there is a second type of cartilage called *meniscal cartilage*. Menisci are pieces of gristle that give extra stability and cushioning to the joint. In the case of the knee, the wrong type of motion can tear this piece of gristle. This typically results in the most common type of cartilage injury— a meniscus tear—but the same event can also injure the surface cartilage. Both types of cartilage have a poor nerve and blood supply and therefore little ability to heal once injured.

In a healthy knee, all of the structures—bone, surface cartilage, meniscal cartilage, muscles, tendons, ligaments, bursa, and skin—work together in a beautiful symphony of motion. Unfortunately, when any part of the orchestra is

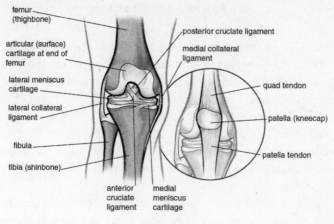

femur
(thighbone)

articular (surface)
cartilage at end of
femur

lateral meniscus
cartilage

lateral collateral
ligament

fibula

tibia (shinbone)

posterior cruciate ligament

medial collateral
ligament

quad tendon

patella (kneecap)

patella tendon

anterior
cruciate
ligament

medial
meniscus
cartilage

Knee anatomy

damaged, it can affect the function of the entire joint. Damage to a ligament causes instability and undue pressure on the cartilage. A tear of the meniscus can cause inflammation and a sense of locking with some movements. A pulled muscle limits motion and thus can cause scarring of other structures. The list of possible maladies can be long, but the treatment of most is the same: Repair the injured structure and proceed to regain full range of motion, strength, coordination, balance, etc.

Pathology

Cartilage Injuries

As discussed earlier, when you hear about someone tearing cartilage, most often that refers to the *meniscal cartilage,* pieces of gristle between the femur and tibia that act as gaskets or spacers (see knee anatomy illustration). Their job is stability, cushioning, and protecting the *surface (articular) cartilage*. Not all meniscal cartilage tears require surgery, but if they cause swelling, catching, and pain, the best chance for a cure is arthroscopy. The surgeon removes the torn bits, or—in a less common situation—throws in some stitches. (A more complete description of arthroscopic surgery comes later in this chapter.)

Damage to the surface (articular) cartilage is called *arthritis*. The suffix *-itis* means "inflammation," as in tendinitis (inflammation of a tendon), arthritis (inflammation of a joint), or bursitis (a bursa is a lubricated sac that allows parts of the body to slide smoothly past one another). When a structure is inflamed, it usually has some combination of pain, swelling, redness, stiffness, and heat. After injury or surgery there is always some inflammation, which I discuss further in Chapter 2.

Arthritis can follow a trauma or can happen simply as a result of age and genetics. Almost everyone over forty has some minor damage to this surface cartilage. Thus, after an unusual stress such as a tough hike or a big spring cleaning, you might get some pain or swelling. Luckily, this usually calms down with rest, ice, and other tricks discussed in Chapter 2. If the knee does not cooperate, the unstable pieces are removed with arthroscopic surgery. The addition of "soft workouts" such as cycling and water exercise to your routine will help keep joints healthy and avoid further damage. Water therapy creates a "natural traction" that pulls apart damaged areas and allows pain-free motion and exercise (see Chapter 9).

In some cases of surface cartilage damage, the surgeon might try to repair it by one of three methods: transferring cartilage from a healthy part of the knee (mosaicplasty), stimulation of new cartilage growth by drilling into the bone marrow (microfracture or multiple drilling), or, finally, actually growing new cartilage in the lab for future transplantation to the knee. These patients often require months on crutches and thus will not begin many of the exercises, movement patterns, and aerobic training immediately after surgery. However, pre-op prep, anti-inflammatory measures, range-of-motion stretches, and crutch walking tips do apply to these surgeries. After the initial recovery from these surface cartilage procedures (usually two to three months), your surgeon will clear you to follow my entire program for total recovery.

ACL and Other Ligament Injuries

The anterior cruciate ligament prevents your femur and tibia bones from sliding past each other—what people used to call a "trick knee" but now call a "blown-out" knee. On any given week during the football or ski season, you will no doubt hear news of athletes who tear their ACL. Because most people who tear their ACL experience this sliding sensation, surgery to reconstruct it is recommended.

The anatomy of the ACL does not allow it to be simply sewn together after it tears (it would be like trying to attach two mop ends). Orthopedic surgeons thus need to reconstruct the ACL, often with tendons borrowed from another part of your own body. This is called an *autograft*. This may sound like a bad idea, but it actually works quite well. The surgeon can use either a strip of your patella tendon (from the injured knee or from the opposite knee) or two small hamstring tendons. A third choice is to use tendons from a dead person, which is called a cadaver graft or *allograft*. Your surgeon will describe the risks and benefits of each of these options, and together you will decide which graft choice is better for you.

Two ligament injuries that do not usually need surgery are tears in the *medial collateral ligament* (MCL) or *posterior cruciate ligament* (PCL). The MCL, the most commonly injured ligament in the knee, heals on its own 95 percent of the time. PCL injuries are much less common than ACL or MCL injuries. Generally, if the PCL is the only ligament torn, you can recover to the point of doing most of your activities and avoid a trip to the operating room.

Severe Arthritis

If you have severe or "end-stage" or "bone-on-bone" arthritis, your doctor might suggest a total knee replacement. The knee is not really "replaced," but the worn joint cartilage is cut away and capped with metal and plastic, much like capping a tooth.

Having an arthritic knee is not a reason to have a TKR. If your knee simply asks for ibuprofen once a week, you do not warrant a trip to the operating room (regardless of what things might look like on your X-ray!). To decide if it might be time to have this procedure on your arthritic knee, ask yourself the following questions: Is knee pain keeping me up at night? Am I dreading the next ball game or graduation because of the walking involved? Does the laundry pile up because I don't want to climb down the stairs to the basement? If the answers to these questions are yes, it might be time to consider a TKR. Perhaps another question that can help you make your decision is: How much do I complain about my knee to the people in my life? Ask them for their input. Life is too short to live with a miserable knee (or with someone who has one).

To recap: Torn meniscal cartilage, ACL injuries, and severe arthritis are the three major maladies indicating surgery and subsequently the rehabilitation program outlined in this book. There are some types of knee procedures, such as cartilage replacement and multiple ligament reconstructions, that would need modifications to this program. One of your doctor's jobs is to make sure you understand just how much the entire process will disrupt your life. Ask questions and arm yourself with as much information as possible.

SURGERY

Arthroscopic Knee Surgery

Except for TKR, almost all other knee surgery involves the arthroscope for at least some part of the procedure. *Arthro* refers to joints, and the *scope* is just a stick about the size of a pencil that contains a fiber-optic light. We attach a camera to one end, allowing the image of the inside of your knee to be projected on a TV screen. When the scope is used, salt water (saline solution) is pumped into your knee to allow the surgeon to move the camera safely and see the various knee structures.

Through another portal or "keyhole" poked in the knee, instruments are inserted that remove any damaged cartilage, put in stitches, drill holes, and so forth. Your surgeon will describe what was done at your first post-op appointment with the help of models and photographs.

The process of pumping up the knee with saline, all by itself, causes the knee to be upset. Because of this trauma, even a high-level athlete will be out for a few weeks after arthroscopic surgery, even if only minor damage was found in the knee.

Doctors describe anterior cruciate ligament surgery as being "arthroscopically aided" since after the small arthroscopic portals are established, longer incisions are also made to drill bone tunnels that will contain the new graft. This extra work makes ACL surgery more traumatic to your knee and thus lengthens the recovery period, making a proper rehab program even more important.

Total Knee Replacement

Most TKRs, on the other hand, are done through a reasonably long incision down the center of your knee, allowing the surgeon to move the kneecap and get to all the surface cartilage. This is definitely *not* "keyhole" surgery. This is the most aggressive of the common knee operations and is the reason why most patients spend up to a week in the hospital afterward. Some surgeons are now doing what is called a "mini-incision" TKR, but it is still major surgery and does not change the program for recovery outlined in this book.

Do I Really Need Surgery?

People often assume that if their knee is swollen and painful, they need surgery to get it fixed. This is simply not the case. As I mentioned earlier, there are many knee injuries—including torn knee cartilage, mild arthritis, and some ligament sprains—that often calm down on their own with the appropriate nonsurgical treatments. As a result, orthopedic surgeons do not sharpen their knives the minute someone enters the office. They might order X-rays to make sure there is no bone damage. Occasionally a magnetic resonance image (MRI) is obtained so the doctor can take a look at the soft tissues (ligaments, tendons, and cartilage) that cannot be seen on an X-ray. After most knee injuries, doctors discuss ways to make the knee feel better (described in the following chapters), recommend home exercises or formal physical therapy, and schedule a follow-up exam. The doctor might also recommend an anti-inflammatory like Advil or Aleve. These medicines help decrease swelling and pain. (For a more detailed discussion of this topic, see Chapter 6.)

As long as you can fully straighten (extend) and fully bend (flex) your knee, you can let it "declare itself." In other words, if it seems to be getting better, you can hold off on any operation. There are lots of folks out there with torn or damaged cartilage who are doing just fine. Again, it is the rare person over forty who does not have *some* cartilage damage. MRI reports are not a reason to have knee surgery. A painful knee with a repairable problem is.

This might be a good time to mention another unhappy aspect of injuring your knee: It usually costs money. Luckily, with most insurance schemes, once you meet your deductible (and you will almost always meet your deductible with any significant problem) insurance will cover 80 percent or more of your expenses. This includes X-rays, MRIs, physical therapy, braces, and so on. Some insurances will also help with the cost of health clubs, personal training, exercise equipment, massage therapy, shoe inserts, etc., with a prescription from your doctor. Get familiar with what paperwork you need, whether from your primary care doctor or orthopedic doctor. A little research and a couple of phone calls up front could save you significant grief later.

[Just as you should not have surgery until your knee is ready, you should not have surgery until your mind is ready. No matter what part of your knee is damaged, doctors still call knee surgery "elective," that is, it can usually be done when it fits into your life. I routinely schedule surgery months in advance to correspond to the end of summer, school vacation, or even just to be ready for ski season. The important thing is to come to the operating room firing on all cylinders, physically and mentally. If you're worried about work or your kid's soccer game, you won't give your knee the attention it deserves. Schedule your surgery when you can dedicate the time and energy it needs to get better. This usually means completely clearing your calendar for at least one week for a knee arthroscopy, three weeks for an anterior cruciate ligament reconstruction, and two months for a total knee replacement.]

As I mentioned, when it comes to your body there is no such thing as "minor" surgery. Furthermore, there is no such thing as minor surgery if it involves a trip to the hospital and an anesthetic. These are significant stressors on your mind and body, and you want to—and need to—prepare for them. There are certain details of your surgery that are beyond the scope of this book, but that doesn't mean that you should not understand the planned procedure. The more you know, the easier it will be for you and the medical staff. Ask questions! Injuring your knee, having surgery, dealing with hospitals, and living with a scar (and possibly metal parts) for the rest of your life are not things we look forward to. They are, however, better than the alternative, which is to give in to your disability and end up on the sidelines watching other people being active and having fun. I cannot stress enough how important it is that you take an active role in your surgery and rehabilitation. The road you are taking is one you must endure for your own sake, but it's not one you have to travel alone. Every page in this book is designed to help you get better faster and with less pain. Take this "portable knee doctor" along as your guide.

GETTING YOUR KNEE READY FOR SURGERY

Decreasing Inflammation
plus Eight Range-of-Motion Stretches
for Before and After Surgery

WHETHER YOUR KNEE is injured from age, trauma, or an operation, the way you take care of it is the same: Decrease the inflammation and regain your motion. Everything else that leads to a healthy knee—balance, coordination, strength, etc.—will follow once you do these two things. As far as your knee is concerned, arthritis = injury = surgery, and this is why we treat them all the same.

Before surgery you must work hard to get the knee in shape. Why? Because you want the surgeon to be working on a knee that is as strong, flexible, and unswollen as possible. For the ligament injury and meniscal tear folks in particular, these criteria speed up post-op pain reduction and recovery. You want to go in to the operating room in the best shape possible, just like an athlete prepared for an event. *You will not recover faster by rushing into surgery*.

For those with long-term arthritis, having good motion and no swelling is a dream, but the message is the same. It may seem counterintuitive to exercise the knee that will soon be "fixed," but the better shape your knee is in going into the operating room, the smoother the rehab road afterward.

RICE

No matter what ails your knee, the initial way to make it feel better is the same: RICE. RICE stands for rest, ice, compression, and elevation and should be used after injury and throughout the course of your rehabilitation. Inflammation (redness, heat, swelling, pain, and stiffness) is the enemy of the knee and is decreased by RICE.

R = Rest

The most obvious way to give your knee rest is to lie down and put some pillows under your leg. Most of us, however, do not have the luxury or the desire to stay off our feet for an extended period of time. Another way to rest the knee, and one that still allows you to get out of the house, is to use crutches. Using crutches does not mean the scary balancing act you sometimes see people attempting. When using crutches properly, you want to put just enough weight on the injured leg to provide balance but not so much as to cause pain. Because we hate to see you limp and get in bad walking habits, doctors usually discourage using only one crutch or a cane. Whether you put ten pounds (what doctors consider "touch-down weight-bearing") or one hundred pounds on that foot, you should perform a left-right gait to mimic normal walking. (Crutch walking is covered in more detail in Chapter 4.)

If you live in the North Country, consider spending a few extra dollars to get crampons for the bottoms of your crutches

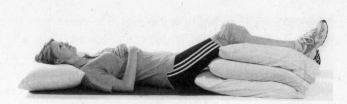

Knee iced and elevated

(see Resources). They are available at most drugstores and may save you from both the embarrassment of falling on the ice and the pain from aggravating the knee even more—or injuring another part of your body.

I = Ice

A big slushy bag of ice that wraps around the knee is terrific for easing pain and swelling. Options for ice include commercial gel packs, a freezer-size plastic bag of crushed ice, frozen peas, or even snow (one good thing about working in New Hampshire is there is a ready supply from November through April—sometimes September through June!).

Apply the ice for twenty minutes at a time with some material (like a washcloth, or put the ice bag in a pillowcase) between the ice bag and your knee so you do not freeze your skin. Do this about every two hours. Keep the knee elevated while you are icing.

C = Compression

Compression can be dangerous unless you are experienced or know someone knowledgeable who can wrap your knee properly. The safest way to add compression by yourself is to wear a long stocking so you are compressing from the toes all the way up to the groin. You can find these stockings (a popular brand is T.E.D.) in most pharmacies (see Resources). In a pinch, a set of supportive tights is better than nothing. Ace bandages are great to hold on ice bags but avoid wrapping them around just the knee, as this can cause swelling below the wrap. If you do use an Ace bandage, use at least two and start from the toes, wrapping your entire leg.

Another way to reduce swelling is to add massage to the mix. Put some oil or lotion on your hands and knead the swelling up toward your thigh so it can drain to your heart. All of your bodily fluids must eventually get to the heart so they can be pumped to their next destination. Try to elevate your knee while you are doing this. Right after surgery you can massage over the stocking. Once the stitches are out, you can gently massage the wound, but do not pull apart the incision as it could make for an uglier scar. (For more on massaging your post-op knee, see Chapter 6.)

E = Elevation

When it comes to elevation, a footstool won't do. The key to proper elevation is getting your knee above your heart. With really nasty swelling, you can lie on the floor with your leg propped up against the wall (just stop before your foot gets numb!). If you are at work, sitting at a desk with your foot on a chair is better than nothing, but it is not complete elevation. One thing is certain: Getting on an airplane or going for a long car ride—where you cannot elevate the knee at all—is just about the worst thing you can do during the two weeks after a knee injury or surgery.

GET IT MOVING

The following movements are designed to be done both *before and after surgery*. I've broken them down into two separate groups: range-of-motion stretches (ROMs) and strengthening exercises (shown in Chapter 3). Getting back your full range of motion—that is, being able to fully straighten and bend your knee—is the first key to getting the knee ready for the operating room. *If you do nothing else, work hard on these range-of-motion stretches both before and after surgery.*

Before you begin the program, use the Basic Equipment Checklist to assemble everything you will need to allow your stretching and exercise sessions to flow.

Basic Equipment Checklist

Regardless of what they say on the infomercials, you can get superstrong using low-tech equipment. These items are simple to obtain and are just as effective as the machines and apparatus you find in an expensive health club. Here is a list of some basics to have available for your rehab.

Got It:

[   ] A television

Much as it pains me to say it, a TV while you're recovering from injury is a key component to both entertain and distract you. A lot of rehab is just plain boring, so I am in favor of anything that keeps you engaged while doing it.

[   ] A chair

[   ] A towel

[   ] Two or three firm pads or pillows

[   ] A strong kitchen table or workout bench

Make It:

[   ] Saddlebag / purse weights

To make a saddlebag weight, throw a couple of two liter soda bottles, weights (easily found at Wal-Mart, local hardware stores, or eBay), or other heavy objects in some old socks. Tie them together so you can hang the saddlebag on your knee or ankle for passive stretches. An old purse, with a towel padding the straps, also works well. The saddlebag or purse should live under your couch or wherever you spend time sitting so you can pop it on obsessively. Multitask by hanging the saddlebag or purse just below or on top of an ice bag surrounding your knee. To be effective, your saddlebag or purse should weigh 10 to 15 pounds.

[ ] Ice, in abundance, at all times

Want It:

[ ] Ankle weights
These will help get you stronger and are available at any sporting goods store.

[ ] Dumbbells
These too will help you get stronger and are also widely available.

[ ] Stability ball
Also known as an exercise ball, physioball, or balance ball, this item is such a great piece of exercise equipment that I think everyone should have one. This adds balance and coordination to your rehab program as you get to the more advanced exercises.

[ ] Access to a swimming pool
Water is simply the safest and most effective place to do the movement pattern prong of your recovery. (Your three-pronged attack of rehabilitation is discussed more in the next chapter.)

[ ] An indoor bicycle or your outdoor bicycle on an indoor trainer
A trainer is a device that your outdoor bike screws into allowing you to ride it indoors. Any bike you ride needs to be properly fitted at a qualified bike shop.

[ ] Water noodle or other flotation device
If you can't find the above equipment locally, check Resources at the end of this book.

Eight Range-of-Motion Stretches

You should do range-of-motion stretches, or ROMs, your entire life to keep your body limber and ready for action. As a result, you will be doing these eight stretches not only pre-op and post-op, but also as part of all of the programs in this book (so get used to them!). They should become old friends over time. You may already recognize some of them from gym class or sessions at the physical therapist's office. Do your stretches and exercises with both legs, starting with the healthier knee.

When going through your stretching and exercise routine, do all the movements with your well leg first and then the injured leg. This serves a few purposes. First, well-leg exercises allow your brain to figure out the movement on a normal knee and then translate that knowledge to the injured knee. Well-leg exercises coupled with upper-body exercises, can help keep your sanity by allowing you an aggressive strength and cardio workout. The resulting increased blood flow also helps pump the swelling out of the injured knee. Finally, well-leg, upper-body, or core exercises (sit-ups, etc.) can serve as a good warm-up before doing your knee exercise program.

TWO RULES FOR STRETCHING AND EXERCISING

1. *Breathe.* People tend to hold their breath on the exertion part of an exercise. That makes the movement more difficult and isn't good for you anyway. Exhale on the exertion and inhale with the relaxation. For example, when doing a sit-up, exhale as you sit up and inhale as you lower your torso down. This also sets up a rhythm for your movements.

Proper breathing has a big effect when you stretch. As you stretch, exhale slowly all the way. Hold the
(continued)

stretch and inhale. Then exhale and stretch some more. You'll see that exhaling allows the muscle to stretch farther.

2. *Strengthen your "core."* As soon as your knee started to hurt, you probably began to walk differently, favoring one leg over the other, limping, putting your feet in odd positions, anything to ease the pain. This can lead to pain in other parts of your body: your opposite knee, your hips, your back—everything gets thrown out of whack. Having a strong core—that is, strong hip, back, and abdominal muscles—will help avoid some of these issues. We talk about this later, but for now, try doing all your exercises with strong, contracted abs. A strong core not only helps you keep good form during standing exercises, but is something to strive for while gardening, shoveling snow, indeed for all of your daily activities.

EXTENSION STRETCHES

PASSIVE EXTENSIONS

Purpose: The first step in prepping for surgery and recovering from any knee injury or surgery is getting the knee moving through a full range of motion. This means being able to fully straighten it (extension) and fully bend it (flexion). Extension is

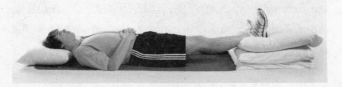

Passive extension

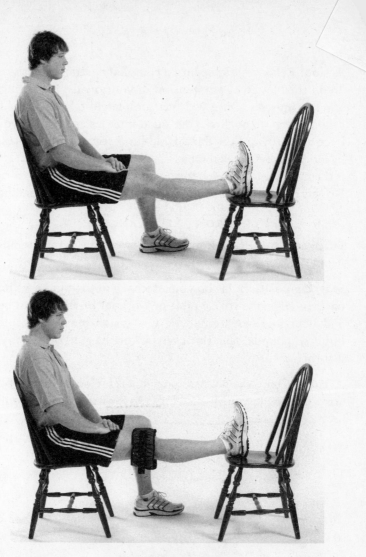

Passive extension with weight

usually the tougher of the two for ACL reconstructions, while bending is generally tougher for TKRs and knee arthroscopies.

Starting position: Lie on your back with your heel propped on a firm pillow or stool, or sit with your heel on a chair or edge of a coffee table. To increase the stretch, drape your saddlebag/purse over your knee.

Action: Relax your knee into a completely straight position. To do this, let go of any tension in your quads, hamstrings, and hip muscles. Once you feel completely relaxed, periodically tighten up or "fire" your quad muscles as you pull your knee *down* toward the floor. Hold for 5 seconds, then relax.

Do passive extension for at least 15 minutes each hour. This is the most critical stretch to do in the first two weeks post-op. Do this habitually, whether you are lying, sitting, or standing.

PRONE LEG HANGS

Purpose: To further promote *full* extension (straightening) using the weight of your lower leg.

Starting position: Lie on your stomach with your knees just past the edge of a strong table or workout bench or your bed and your legs out straight. If you weigh more than three hundred pounds, save this exercise for the gym or the physical therapy area.

Action: Completely relax your muscles and feel a good stretch through your hamstrings. As a variation, have some-

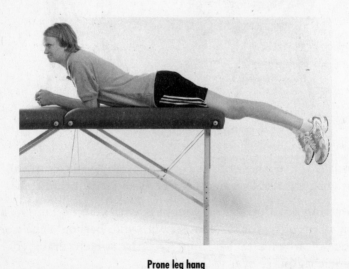

Prone leg hang

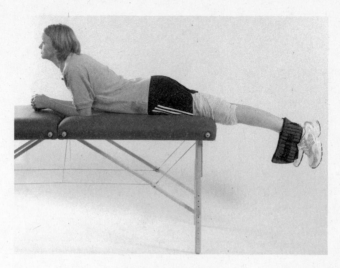

Prone leg hang with weight

one hang the saddlebag or purse on your ankle and put a hot wet towel on your hamstring for further relaxation. Hang for 5–10 minutes, not just a few seconds.

CAT WALK POSE

Purpose: To promote *full* extension in a standing position.

Starting position: Stand with your good leg fully extended and the other leg slightly bent.

Action: Gradually tighten your quadriceps and gently push your knee backward to attain full straightening. If you are standing and talking to someone or waiting in line, strike this pose. It is exactly what your injured knee does *not* want to do, but do it anyway!

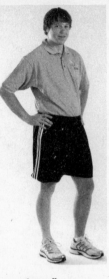

Cat walk pose

STANDING FULL EXTENSION

Purpose: To achieve full straightening and hamstring flexibility.

Starting position: Stand with your injured leg propped on a table or chair with your knee completely straight.

Action: Press down firmly on your thigh as you lean forward to stretch your hamstring. Bend the standing knee to increase the stretch. Perform for 30–60 seconds, 5 times on each leg. Since this is an aggressive stretch, start with your heel on a stair or low chair to ease into the movement.

TOWEL STRETCHES

Purpose: To get the knee as straight as possible—at least as straight as your uninjured knee.

Starting position: Sit on a bench, bed, chair, or the floor.

Action: Wrap a towel (or a long scarf) around the ball of your foot, holding the ends. Pull toward you, keeping your knee down and thus lifting your foot off the surface. You should feel a good stretch in your hamstrings, calf, and

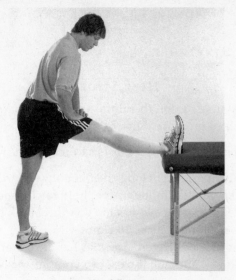

Standing full extension

behind the knee. As with all ROM stretches, give a slow, steady pull and with each exhale feel your muscles stretching a bit farther. Do this exercise as frequently as possible. Just like your saddlebag/purse, your towel should never be out of arm's reach for the weeks pre-op and post-op.

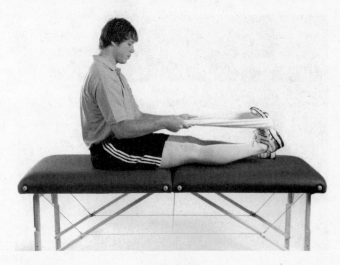

Towel stretch

FLEXION STRETCHES

HEEL SLIDES

Purpose: Active flexion (bending) and extension (straightening) stretch to promote range of motion at the knee.

Starting position: Lie on your back on a flat surface.

Action: Slide your heel along the floor, up toward your buttocks. When you feel mild tension, hold for 1 minute and try to stretch a bit farther. Now, slide your heel back down until your leg is straight. Repeat 10 times.

For an increased stretch, use your hands to grab your shin (*not* your knee!) and pull it closer to your buttocks.

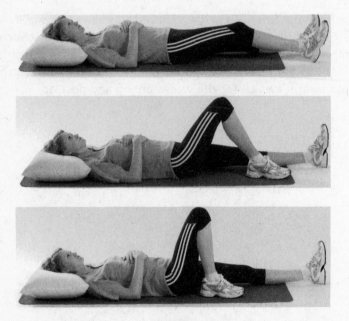

Heel slide

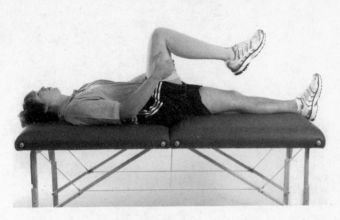

Supine leg hang

SUPINE LEG HANGS

Purpose: To improve your knee's bending ability. It is a passive flexion (bending) exercise.

Starting position: Lie on your back with your knee bent. Clasp your hands behind your thigh.

Action: Relax all your muscles and allow your knee to bend while holding your thigh. Hold for 2 minutes, letting gravity do its thing; then slowly straighten your knee out again. Repeat 5 times.

The key is to relax your muscles. If the straightening feels hard, roll onto your oppisite side and straighten your knee in that position. Then roll onto your back for the next 2-minute supine leg hang.

STANDING FLEXION—FORWARD AND BACKWARD

Purpose: A great stretch to get your knee bending like it is supposed to.

Starting position—forward: Place your foot on a table or chair. The table or chair should be on carpeting or against a wall so it won't move.

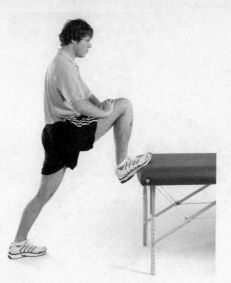

Standing flexion forward

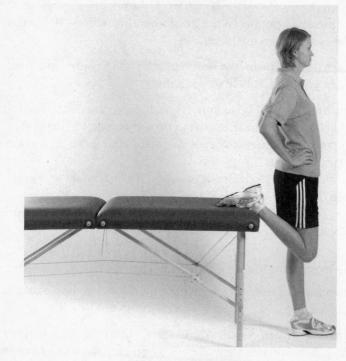

Standing flexion backward

Action: Slowly lean forward, allowing your knee to rest periodically before leaning and stretching a bit more. Hold this position for at least 2 minutes, preferably longer. Gravity is doing all the work, not you, so *relax*.

Starting position—backward: Stand with your back to a table or other stationary object.

Action: Place your foot on the edge of the table. Use your hands to help you get into position. Gently lean or sit back, toward your heel. You are in complete control of how much pressure you want to place on the knee. Do not force it! Hold this position 2 minutes; release; repeat 3 or more times.

Again, the key is to relax your muscles while you strive for more motion. The goal is to touch your heel to your buttocks.

Variation: Kneeling on pillows with a few more pillows under your thighs to prevent flexing too far before you're ready. Slowly ease down, hold for 2–3 minutes, then repeat.

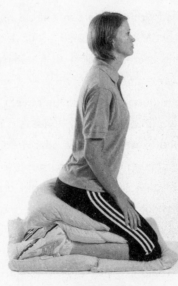

Sitting flexion

Remember, all of these stretches are probably best done in front of a TV or other distraction so that you aren't tempted to rush!

SMART Goal Setting

As you think about your upcoming surgery, make time to set some goals for your recovery. The SMART system is a well-known goal setting guide, introduced by Franklin Covey and used by athletes and businesspersons alike. It stands for:

Specific

Measurable

Achievable

Realistic

Time Phased

Prior to surgery, I want you to concentrate especially on the T, the time aspect of SMART goal setting. I have discovered that most of my patients secretly think their friends who have had knee operations are wimps and that they themselves will fly through surgery and get right back to their lives. While this may occasionally be true (in both cases!), there is a certain amount of basic biology that must take place after an operation. Thus, having the goal of coming back from surgery "faster" than anyone else is not only unrealistic, it's potentially dangerous.

Having a goal of coming back from surgery a better athlete, however, is realistic. For nonathletes, coming back from surgery is an opportunity to become more fit than you have ever been. For now, I would like you to set a long-range goal (one year) and two short-range goals (two and four months). Your process goals, which you should be reaching daily and weekly (including the ROMs, level A exercises, and so forth), are enumerated throughout the book.

Goal setting is much more effective if you commit it to writing. So grab a pencil and fill in the blanks below. In the weeks and months that follow, look back at your goals and jot down new ones as you meet your targets. Remember: Goals do not just happen if you wait two or twelve months. Goals are achieved because you perform each stretch and exercise to your maximum every time.

My Long-Range Goal (where I'd like to be—physically and mentally—in 1 year):

_____

_____

My Short-Range Goal:
2 months after knee surgery:

_____

4 months after knee surgery:

_____

TEN ESSENTIAL
EXERCISES FOR
BEFORE AND AFTER
SURGERY

Prong 1 of the Three-Pronged Attack

As you achieve full range of motion with the stretches from Chapter 2, you can also work toward getting your muscles strong. Having your knee supple and fit *before* surgery makes getting into the house, driving the car, and walking on crutches that much easier *after* surgery. Also, by practicing these exercises, you establish a smooth highway between your brain, spinal cord, and knee, allowing a seamless transition to more advanced movements (otherwise known as your normal life).

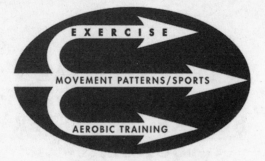

EXERCISE

MOVEMENT PATTERNS/SPORTS

AEROBIC TRAINING

LEVEL A EXERCISES

Exercises represent the first prong of my three-pronged attack toward getting your knee healthy. For those who have not darkened the door of a gym for a while, enlist a friend who can read the text aloud and help you match your body position with the photos. If you are an active, athletic person, the exercises should seem simple. Their purpose, however, is to educate your muscles so you can move on to more aggressive training. Remember: Trying to get back too quickly from an injury sometimes results in more, not less, time off.

QUAD SETS

Purpose: Your quadriceps muscle, the big muscle on the front of your thigh, takes any opportunity to go on vacation

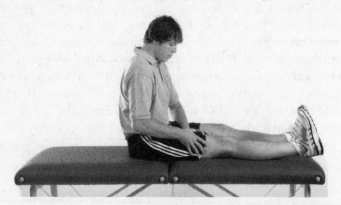

Quad set

after knee trauma. As a result, do quad sets on your way into surgery and make them the first thing you do in the recovery room. Quad sets are truly a key exercise everyone should do for any lower-extremity problem.

Starting position: Lying down, sitting on the floor, or standing, begin with your leg straight.

Action: Tighten your quadriceps muscle and hold for 5 seconds. If you are sitting or lying, pull the back of your knee *down* so your leg actually bends backward as far as it can ("back knee" or "hyperextended"). While you pull your knee down, lift your foot up and toward you. The feeling in the back of your knee should be similar to when you do the towel stretch illustrated in the previous chapter. Do 3 sets of 5 reps and hold each rep for 5 seconds. Attempt to increase the quad contraction during these 5 seconds.

Perform these exercises at work, in class, or at home, multiple times a day. People who do Pilates can think of quad sets as the knee version of an abdominal contraction. Your first motion is *down,* pressing your knee into the floor, similar to pulling in your stomach muscles. The second motion is the quad contraction, similar to raising your chest with your stomach pulled in.

WHAT ARE REPS AND SETS?

A rep is a repetition of a particular exercise. A set is a group of repetitions. Thus, 3 sets of 5 reps is a total of 15 exercises. The other way to do exercises is by time. For example, do quad sets of 5 seconds, followed by 5 seconds of rest, for 2 minutes. The benefit of doing exercises by time is you do not rush trying to finish a predetermined number of reps. Whatever your method, strive to do all exercises slowly, carefully, and deliberately.

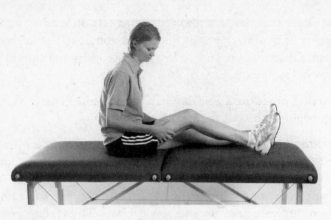

Hamstring set

HAMSTRING SETS

Purpose: To increase control and strength of the hamstrings, that wad of muscles on the back of your thigh. For ACL patients, the hamstring is the muscle that works in concert with the ligament to stabilize the forward motion of the tibia bone. (For those with normal ACLs, strong hamstrings help keep them that way.)

Starting position: Lying down or sitting, begin with your leg bent.

Action: Tighten your hamstring muscles by pushing down and back (toward you) on your heel, and hold for 5 seconds. Do 3 sets of 5 reps and hold each rep for 5 seconds. Attempt to increase the contraction during these 5 seconds by pulling steadily harder. Watch out for cramps. Perform these exercises at work, in class, or at home, several times a day.

CO-CONTRACTIONS

Purpose: This is another one of those critically important exercises that you will be doing obsessively. When you simultaneously contract the quadriceps (front of the thigh) and

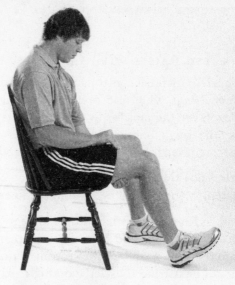

Co-contraction

hamstrings (in back of the thigh), your knee is stabilized. Co-contraction means muscles contracting together—something that needs to take place automatically, as this stability serves to protect your knee ligaments and cartilage (thus well worth practicing).

Starting position: Sit on a chair. Bend your lower leg so that it forms a 90-degree angle with your thigh. (If your chair is too high, put a dictionary on the floor under your foot.)

Action: Contract both your hamstring and quadriceps muscle by pushing your heel into the floor and pulling backward at the same time. Your foot does not move. This takes a bit of practice, but it is important that you master this. Place your hands on the front and back of your thigh so you can feel the muscles tighten. Do the well leg first so your brain knows what you're trying to accomplish on the injured leg. Do 3 sets of 5 reps and hold each rep for 5 seconds. Attempt to increase the contraction during these 5 seconds by pulling steadily harder. Breathe!

LEG RAISES WITH CO-CONTRACTION

Purpose: To increase control and strength of the quadriceps and hamstrings, while also strengthening the hip flexors. The hip flexors are the muscles in your groin that bend your hip, lifting the thigh bone toward your chest. This is also a great "core" exercise as it also works your abdominal muscles.

Starting position: Begin with your leg co-contracted (lying or seated) with a 30-degree bend in the knee.

Action 1: Keeping your leg in this 30-degree position, lift it 2 feet off the floor. Hold for 5 seconds, then lower your leg back to the floor. Maintain the co-contraction, keeping those quad and hamstring muscles working hard throughout the movement. Do 2 sets of 5 reps on each side and hold each rep for 5 seconds.

Action 2: Co-contract and raise and lower the leg quickly without touching it down to the floor. Do 2 sets of 10 reps on each side. Try to perform one rep every second.

Challenge: Once you feel strong enough, you can do this exercise (and others as noted) with ankle weights. Start with two to three pounds on each ankle and progress up from there. Perform this exercise at least two times per day.

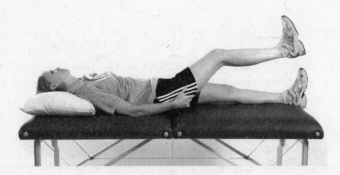

Leg raise with co-contraction

PRONE HAMSTRING CURLS

Purpose: To increase control and strength of the hamstrings through an active range of motion. This is a tough but important exercise for you hamstring ACL patients. Don't worry! Time and perseverance will win out.

Starting position: Lie on your stomach, legs straight.

Action: Bend your knee by bringing your heel as close to your gluteals (buttocks) as possible, then lower your leg with a slow, smooth, *controlled* motion. Do this exercise slowly. Count slowly to 4 going up, and count to 4 again going down. Do 2 sets of 10 reps on each side, twice a day.

Challenge: Add ankle weights after gaining control and strength.

Bonus: As you get better at this exercise, try lifting the thigh and knee off the floor before starting the hamstring curl. This really works the buttocks muscles, as again strong hips are another key to strong knees.

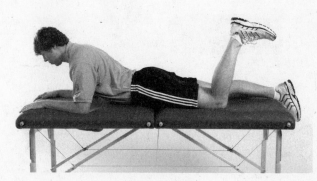

Prone hamstring curl

HEEL RAISES

Purpose: To increase strength in your calf muscles and get a good stretch in the back of your leg.

Starting position: Standing. Hold onto a chair back or the wall for balance.

Action: Slowly rise up on to your toes, hold, and return to the starting position. Do 2 sets of 10 reps, twice a day. Since the only apparatus you need is legs, you can do this exercise anywhere—waiting for the bus, riding in an elevator, at the sink while washing dishes, etc.

Challenge: Stand on the edge of a stair, with the balls of your feet on the stair and your heels unsupported. Rise, then lower down as far as you can, below the level of the step. (If you don't

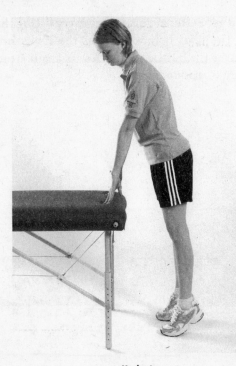

Heel raise

have stairs in your home, stand on a dictionary.) Or perform the exercise one leg at a time. Think balance!

Warning: This simple exercise can be surprisingly hard if you go slow and use the full range of ankle motion. You may have to work up to the suggested number of reps.

Positive Self-Talk

[While most of us are quick to give others a pat on the back, we rarely do the same for ourselves. Positive self-talk (repeating affirming words or phrases or simply saying something nice about yourself) can be another tool in your recovery. Keeping a positive attitude is not always easy—there may be pain and setbacks throughout the process. Sometimes all we need is a minor attitude adjustment to get past such moments. Positive self-talk can do just that.

Try coming up with one or two mantras you can repeat during tough times. A positive word might be "strong" or "tough" or "unstoppable." Examples of positive phrases are:

I will not let this beat me.

I have a high pain tolerance.

I'm on the road to recovery.

Create two or three self-talk words or statements of your own. Write them somewhere readily visible to establish their power.]

HIP EXTENSIONS

Purpose: To get great gluts and strengthen your lower back.

Starting position: Lie on your stomach. You can place a pillow under your hips to decrease stress on your back.

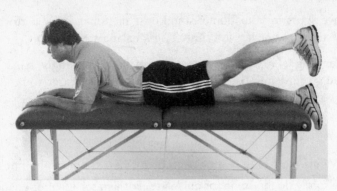

Hip extension

Action: Lift your leg just off the floor with the knee straight. Squeeze the buttock for 3 seconds. Slowly lower your leg, always in control. Raise (and lower) the opposite hand straight out in front of you at the same time. Do 2 sets of 10 reps at least once a day. It's okay if you can't raise your leg far. As long as your thigh is supporting itself, you're doing fine.

Challenge: Add ankle weights when you're ready.

DOUBLE-LEG SQUATS

Purpose: *Squats are the cornerstone functional exercise for your legs.* Almost every sport has its players in a partial squat a large percentage of the time. Watch any football, soccer, baseball, tennis, or basketball player or snowboarder as he or she assumes the "ready position." This is simply a quarter squat with the arms held out (see photo).

Starting position: Begin with your feet shoulder width apart. Hold onto a chair or other secure object.

Action: Squat as if you are sitting down in a chair. Keep your lower back straight and strong. You may eventually go as low as 90 degrees but start by doing quarter squats to 45 degrees, or as low as you can comfortably go. Do 2 sets of 10 reps, twice a day.

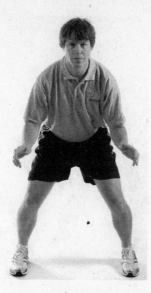

Ready position

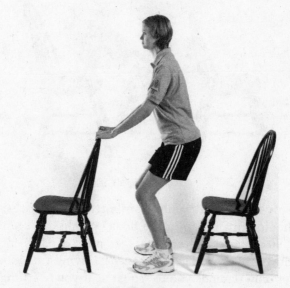

Double-leg squat

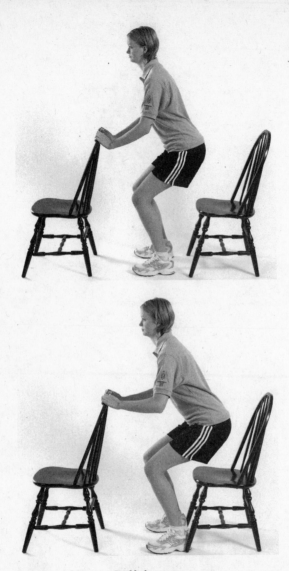

Double-leg squats

Keep your weight evenly distributed on both legs. Your feet should remain flat on the floor. As you can see in the photo, 90 degrees is a deep squat, and most of us do not need to go down this low to get the benefit. Having a chair behind you not only reminds you to "squat as if you're sitting" but also can serve as a bail out if you get fatigued.

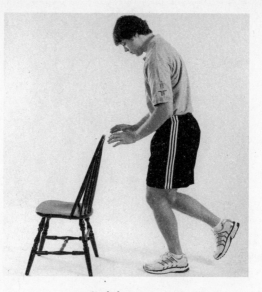

Single-leg stance

SINGLE-LEG STANCE

Purpose: To improve balance, increase strength, and develop proprioception—a sixth sense radar system that simply means knowing where your body is in space (without having to look). Having good balance and becoming aware of how your body is positioned at any given moment will give you a tremendous advantage in preventing injuries and falls.

Starting position: Stand with a chair or something stable for balance.

Action: Stand on one leg. Keep the knee of your standing leg slightly bent in a nice, co-contracted position. Hold for 5 seconds after letting go of the chair and work up to 30–60 seconds. Try not to touch the opposite foot to the floor.

Challenge: Close your eyes or stand on a Dyna Disc (see Resources), hard pillow, or something similar to challenge your balance. The single-leg stance is another one of those exercises you should do obsessively, like when waiting in line for Rolling Stones tickets or talking to your broker.

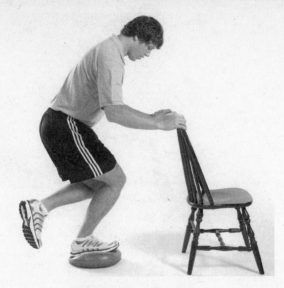

Single-leg stance with Dyna Disc

At this point you might be noticing a pattern. I am asking you to incorporate knee rehab into your life, not just for a specific number of minutes a day. Don't relegate stretching and exercise to the time spent with your therapist or trainer. Those sessions are just the tip of the total recovery iceberg.

QUICK STEP RUNNING

Purpose: Quick step running allows you to "run" soon after surgery by using your calf and hip muscles to absorb the shock. Depending on the state of your knee, even quick steps might be too aggressive to do before surgery, but give it a try, perhaps not so "quickly."

Starting position: Start in the ready position (see page 49). This is the position that many sports start from since it allows you to move quickly in any direction.

Action: Quickly step from one foot to the other. Stay in place, keep your feet close to the ground, and think light and quick. Gain confidence before increasing the speed. Do 3 sets of 30 seconds each, twice a day.

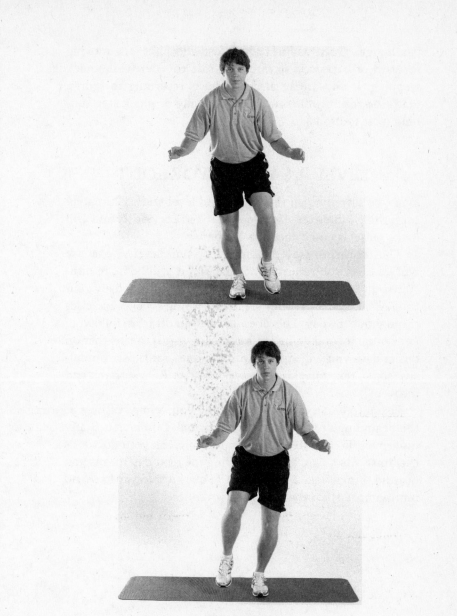

Quick step running

Challenge: Once you're feeling fast and light, try moving forward or backward or laterally (side to side) while quick stepping. If you are an athlete who is returning to sports, your first running outside should actually be quick step running (soft footfalls).

LEVEL A SAMPLE WORKOUT

Don't be scared by all this prong and level stuff. Ultimately everything builds on what you practiced previously and will make sense as you come to it. I promise.

The following table summarizes your Level A exercise workout. As you return to normal life, it will be more difficult to fit blocks of time for your knee into your daily routine. As suggested, get in the habit of doing Level A exercises throughout the day. This does not let you off from following your program and doing your exercises; it just means that on busier days you will still get in some reps. For those compulsive souls, take one day off a week just to ROM stretch and recover.

Listen to what your body is telling you. Some stiffness at the beginning of your workout is normal. Pain is not. If any movement is consistently uncomfortable, ask your doctor or therapist. Also, pain and/or swelling the next day means you overdid things. Take a day off until your knee feels better and limit your reps for the next few workouts.

LEVEL A SAMPLE WORKOUT

EXERCISE	FREQUENCY	COMMENTS
Quad sets	3 sets of 5 reps 2 times a day	• Perform at home, school, work, the office, etc. • Quad sets should become a reflex throughout the day.
Hamstring sets	3 sets of 5 reps 2 times a day	• You can never have hamstrings that are too strong.
Co-contractions	3 sets of 5 reps multiple times a day	• Feel the muscles with your hands.
Leg raises with co-contraction*	2 sets of 5 reps (each side) 2 times a day	• It takes concentration to perform the co-contraction without your foot on the floor.
Prone hamstring curls*	2 sets of 10 reps (each side) 2 times a day	• Slow and steady hamstring ACL patients.
Heel raises*	2 sets of 10 reps 2 times a day	• Use a stair to increase the ROM.
Hip extensions*	2 sets of 10 reps once a day	• Think rock-solid butt.
Double-leg squats	2 sets of 10 reps 2 times a day	• The workhorse exercise you will do the rest of your life.
Single-leg stance	Work up to 60 seconds multiple times a day	• Become obsessive about this move.
Quick step running	3 sets of 30 seconds twice a day	• Feel light, quick, quiet.

*With time, add ankle weights to these exercises for increased strengthening.

THREE WORKOUT RULES TO REMEMBER

1. Stretch. Range-of-motion stretches (Chapter 2) are not just something you do if you have time. They are an integral part of your program. Stretch the appropriate muscle group before and after each exercise, and then do a slightly longer stretch after the full workout as part of your cooldown. Take a look at Chapter 6 for a Sample Day routine, which includes warm-up and cooldown suggestions.

2. Ice. After your workout, ice your knee for 20 minutes with it elevated above your heart. Any increase in swelling or discomfort should alert you to cut back on the exercises and ask your doctor or therapist if you need to make adjustments.

3. Have fun! Do not make doing your exercises torture. Do them in front of the TV or recruit someone to do them with you. (Perhaps you can entice a friend by noting that these exercises might just keep him or her out of the operating room!)

Mental Movies

Preparing your knee for surgery involves gaining full range of motion and waking up the muscles. Getting your mind ready is a bit trickier. One method of mental preparation, most commonly associated with athletes, is imagining or picturing the event in your head. Picturing a strong, mobile knee will help your body understand what you're trying to achieve. We refer to this type of mental preparation as imagery or visualization. Imagery is a simple, enjoyable, and effective tool for speeding your recovery. Good imagery incorporates all senses: taste, touch, sound, smell, and, of course, sight. For your first foray into imagery, use your imaginary senses to produce a mental rehab movie.

Imagine a time before your injury when you felt fit and happy. Picture a hike with your dog, a great day skiing, working in your garden, anything that has you moving on a strong knee. Whatever you choose, it should be an image that defines you and is one you remember and cherish. Next, take fifteen seconds of that image and make it a mental movie you can replay at will. (This will take practice.)

Play your movie clip at any stressful time during your knee adventure. It doesn't matter if the image is recent, but it should be fun, clear, and make you feel strong! As you close your eyes and play your mental movie, try to imagine other senses to make the movie as vivid as possible. Add in the temperature that day, the smell of the grass, or a song that was playing. If you are having trouble with your imagery selection, change the film and find one you like better.

Imagery techniques are employed by top athletes and performers for one very good reason: They work.

GETTING YOUR LIFE READY FOR SURGERY

Pre-op Checklists and Tips—

Sweating the Small Stuff

THE BEST DOCTORS and nurses are compulsive, and so are the best patients. The following suggestions will complement the information you received from your surgeon. Bottom line: For things to go as smoothly as possible, you need to sweat the small stuff!

Three Pre-op Checklists

1. Is Your Kitchen Ready?

Have on hand:

[   ] Vanilla protein powder for shakes, frappés, and smoothies

[ ] Cut-up melon, berries, or other in-season fruits and vegetables

[ ] Cold water, fruit juices, and energy drinks

[ ] Protein bars such as Power, Balance, Luna bars

[ ] Sandwich fixings

[ ] Whole-grain sandwich bread or wraps

[ ] Ice

When you had two good knees, you didn't think twice about squatting to get something out of a low cabinet or standing on a stepladder to get something off a top shelf. Think again. Make sure the things you use every day are within easy reach.

2. Is Your Medicine Cabinet Ready?

Useful items to stock up on:

[ ] Acetaminophen (e.g., Tylenol)

[ ] Ibuprofen or naproxen (e.g., Advil, Aleve)

[ ] Antibiotic ointment (e.g., Bacitracin, neosporin)

[ ] Rubbing alcohol, witch hazel, or peroxide

[ ] Massage oil or lotion containing vitamin E

[ ] Sunblock (SPF 45 or greater) to put on your scars after surgery

[ ] Sterile 4×4 gauze bandages

3. Are *You* Ready for Surgery?

Practical matters to focus on prior to the day of your surgery:

[ ] Are all of your questions answered?

[ ] Have you read your preoperative instructions thoroughly? Is all your paperwork gathered and in order?

[ ] Do you know which hospital or surgical center you are going to?

[ ] Do you know exactly how to get there? (Seriously, guys, do you *really* know how to get there?)

[ ] Do you have someone to drive you? Remember: You will NOT BE ABLE TO DRIVE (physically or legally) or operate machinery as long as you are on narcotic medication.

[ ] Have you heard from the hospital regarding what time you need to be there? (If you haven't, call the operating room nurse at the hospital or check with your doctor's office.)

[ ] Is your stomach empty? Again, it is vital that you DO NOT EAT OR DRINK ANYTHING—not even water—after midnight the night before your surgery. If you eat or drink anything after midnight, your surgery will be canceled. Any type of anesthesia is more dangerous with something in your stomach due to the risk of vomiting.

[ ] The night before surgery, take two acetaminophen (not aspirin!) tablets (if you have no sensitivities to Tylenol) after a shower with antibacterial soap. *Scrub everywhere!* Repeat the shower in the morning, but not the acetaminophen. The fewer bacteria you bring into the operating room, the better.

[ ] After your morning shower, use a magic marker or pen to mark the thigh of the operative knee.

[ ] If you already have crutches, remember to bring them. Be sure to practice your "touch-down" crutch walking (described in this chapter).

[ ] Also bring:

- A Cryo/Cuff or other icing device if you have one. There are numerous commercial icing options; Cryo/Cuff is just one popular brand. Ask your friends who had knee surgery if they have a clean one of these devices you can borrow.

- Any prescription meds you are presently taking.
- A hydrated, rested body and mind.
- The ability to de-stress through conscious breathing (see later in this chapter).
- Some good reading material.
- This book.
- A big smile, knowing you have done everything you can for a positive outcome!

PRE-OP TIPS

Rally Your Support Team

When planning for knee surgery, don't tell friends and family, "I'll call if I need you." *You will need a support team.* For arthroscopies, having someone around for two nights after surgery should suffice. After an ACL reconstruction, plan on help for about a week, and for a TKR, you want help for at least two full weeks after you get home, assuming you are in the hospital for about one week.

When choosing people to help you, ask someone who makes you feel good and who will be a positive addition to your rehab process. You do not need negative energy in the house while you are recovering. Advice from friends is welcome, but if someone starts a sentence with, "When I had my surgery . . ." throw him or her out! Every knee is different. You cannot compare your left knee and right knee much less your surgery with your sister-in-law's. The job of the support team is to ask, "How can I help you?"

Keep Your Body Well Hydrated, Well Nourished

The weeks before and after surgery are not the time to go on a grapefruit diet. You should eat and drink healthful foods, but be sure to stop eating completely by midnight on the night before the operation. A balanced diet should contain plenty of protein, fruits and vegetables, vitamins, minerals, and carbohydrates (yes, carbs). Whether you are hiking a mountain, clearing a field, or having surgery, you need to have energy, and carbohydrates are the simplest form of energy for your body to use.

Hydration is equally important for your pre- and post-op preparation. On the days before and after the operation, you should constantly have diluted juice or diluted energy drink within arm's reach. Getting ready for surgery is no different from preparing for a running or cycling race. You will be putting stresses on your body and want that body to be in the best shape possible to tackle those stresses. Having your nutrients and hydration levels topped off going into surgery is just another part of that preparation. Afterward, you need more hydration to flush the anesthetics and other nasty chemicals out of your system.

Get Rid of the Junk

Here's a simple way to make surgery a positive experience: In the days before your operation, *clear all of the junk food out of your pantry and refrigerator.* All of it. Sugar is like cigarettes: If you don't have any, you don't miss it. But if you have a little, you want more. Replace the junk food with some healthy, low-salt, and low-fat snacks (e.g., low-salt nuts, rice cakes, cut-up fruit, yogurt). Also, throw in some energy bars containing plenty of protein.

You might not have much of an appetite the days after surgery, so any calories you ingest should be worthwhile. Fruits, protein bars, energy drinks, smoothies, healthy shakes, and frappés all give you much-needed nutrients. Have some fruit sliced and easily accessible for a great source of vitamins and water. I also advise patients to take a multivitamin supplement containing iron for at least a month after surgery— longer if you had a TKR, as you will lose more blood than with other knee operations.

New pantry, new knee, new you . . . with only premium fuel going into your recovering engine.

Conscious Breathing

[One way to relax body and mind is to practice conscious breathing. This simply means being aware of the air moving in and out of your lungs. Breathe through your nose and fill your chest from the "bottom up" by using your diaphragm and abdominal muscles. As you exhale, relax all of your muscles, starting with your toes and moving up slowly to your shoulders and neck. Try calling to mind a quiet, relaxing scene from your life, such as looking on a still lake or lying in a hammock.

Conscious breathing is so simple that it's hard at first. We are accustomed to constant stimulation, noise, and interference—from street sounds to cell phones to television. In the weeks leading up to surgery, set aside a few minutes every day to focus on the air as it moves in and out of your body. The ability to do some conscious breathing gives you a lifelong tool for reducing stress, whether you use it before surgery or whenever you're feeling anxious. The mental imagery you were doing earlier should get you excited and feeling strong. Use conscious breathing and some quiet imagery to make you calm.]

Practice Crutch Walking

Try to get hold of a pair of crutches before surgery. Even just five minutes of practice will save you significant grief in the days to come. Be careful of throw rugs, slippery floors, dogs, or small children that can pose a hazard. Most doctors have patients use "touch-down" weight bearing when first using crutches.

HOW TO USE CRUTCHES

Find the Proper Height

- Stand erect with shoes on and shoulders relaxed. There should be a space of about two inches between your armpit and the top of the crutch.

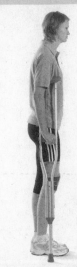

- Support your weight with your hands, elbows slightly bent.

- The tips of the crutches should be about six inches from the outside of your shoes.

- Never lean on your armpits. Keep the top of the crutch against your chest.

Do a Safety Check

- Check the wing nuts periodically—they should always be tight!

- Replace the crutch tips if they are worn out to prevent slipping.

- Special crampon (spiked) tips are available at local drugstores. These are a necessity in wintry conditions (see Resources).

- Take SUPREME care when walking on wet and slippery surfaces! You will do less harm to your knee putting weight on it than if you slip and fall.

(continued)

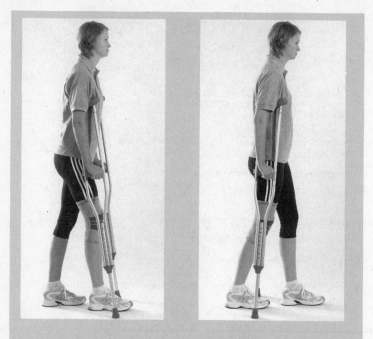

- Ladies, no heels (not even low ones) while using crutches. Wear flat shoes, preferably sneakers.

"Touch-Down" Crutch Walking

- In the same motion, move both crutches and the injured leg ahead in one small step. Touch down for balance (about ten pounds of pressure on the foot) and swing the other leg through to maintain a normal gait pattern. Repeat until you get where you're going.

- Progressively add weight to the involved leg as instructed by your doctor until you are fully weight bearing with confidence.

- Touch-down crutch walking is less stressful to the knee than trying to keep your foot balanced off the ground

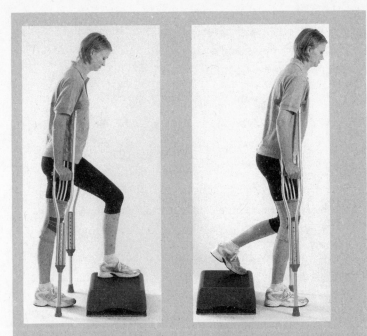

and thus tends to be the least painful way to use crutches. Obviously, any time the knee is dependent (lower than your heart), it can cause some discomfort. If even touch-down weight bearing hurts, it's time to get your knee elevated and iced (see Chapter 2).

Stair Climbing

- The crutches stay on the same level as the involved leg. GO UP A STEP with the uninvolved leg taking the weight. Now bring the crutches and the involved leg up.

- To GO DOWN A STEP, place the crutches down first with the involved leg. Transfer the appropriate weight to the handgrips and lower yourself down onto the uninvolved leg.

(continued)

- If you are unable to go up and/or down stairs on crutches, sit down and go from step to step. This is not pretty, but at least it's safe.

Getting Rid of Your Crutches

- As your knee gets stronger, you should be able to put less and less weight on the crutches and more and more weight on your knee.

- When you feel ready, practice a normal walking pattern in the house, but continue using crutches outside. Ask someone to watch you and make sure you are not limping.

- Crutches are not an all-or-nothing aid. Even if you have not used crutches in the past week, you might still pull them out for a ball game, shopping, or anytime you will be on your feet for an extended period with no chance to rest.

- If you have a busy day and your knee is sore, get back on the crutches for a day to allow your knee to calm down. Remember, crutches are part of the R in RICE.

Practical Matters

The days before surgery should be all about decreasing stress and preparing for surgery. Keep things organized by having a notebook dedicated to all of your medical issues. Write down any questions, answers, phone numbers, contact people, etc. Additionally, have your insurance information and any forms from your doctor's office with you in case there are questions, as you fill out even more paperwork on the day of surgery.

If the hospital is nearby, swing by so you know what entrance you'll be using and where to park. If you have to travel, leave even more time than you think you need—especially if the hospital is in a city. You are going to do plenty of waiting once you get to the hospital, so a few extra minutes to decrease overall stress should be time well spent.

Prepare Your Recovery Bed

Have your recovery bed ready before you leave for surgery to ensure a smooth hospital-to-home transition. This means a firm bed on the ground floor located near a bathroom and away from any steps. This is especially vital for TKR patients. If there is no appropriate bed available, call your health insurance provider to see about renting a hospital bed. If this is not an option, you can place a piece of plywood between the box spring and the mattress. (Creative problem solving generally works best *before* surgery.)

Have some fun hobby items close at hand, like balls, rackets, hand weights, knitting, cards, etc., to keep you sane and happy. They will also keep your hand-to-eye coordination and your visualization (imagery) going. Remember that your therapy will also include practicing movement patterns immediately after surgery. While it is good to have fun distractions nearby, be sure to keep the floor clear for crutch safety!

Shower with an Antibacterial Soap

For everyday use, antibacterial soaps have not been shown to be any more effective than regular soap. For the *night before and the morning of surgery,* however, I advise a good scrub with an antibacterial soap. Use a brush or a clean cloth and scrub *everywhere*. Shampoo your hair. Don't put on any cologne, lotion, nail polish, or other such products. Wear clean, comfortable clothes, including fresh underwear and a loose pair of boxers or gym shorts. Most hospitals allow you to keep your underwear on for knee surgery if it can be pushed up easily.

Put an old stool in the tub or shower, since you will want to sit when your doctor gives the okay to bathe. Put rubber tips, or something else nonskid, on the feet of the stool so it doesn't zoom out from under you.

ARE YOU READY?

Let's review our preparation for surgery: Your knee is as good as it can be. Your family and friends are ready to chip in and help out during the first few days or weeks of your recovery. You do not have anything pressing on your schedule for the coming weeks—no ball games, concerts, trips, meetings, etc. You understand and have practiced the range-of-motion stretches and Level A exercises. You have books, toys, videos, and other items for fun distraction. Finally, you have a healthy pantry and an accessible bed waiting for you when you come home.

You are ready. The stressful decisions have been made. Now the game is on.

THE SURGERY ITSELF

What to Expect

AT THIS POINT, all the hard prep work has been done and decisions made. You are rested, hydrated, and strong. You will not be given any information the day of your operation that has not already been covered. The nurses and doctors realize you are nervous and will do all they can to make you feel comfortable and confident. Any additional information they want you to know will be written down and given to whoever has accompanied you to the hospital.

Remember that doctors and nurses do this every day. Though I said there is no such thing as minor surgery, there is routine surgery, and that is what you want. Routine is how the fewest mistakes are made. It will seem like a dozen people ask you which is the operative knee, if you have any allergies, if you ate anything since midnight, or if you have any major medical problems, because a dozen people will. At the risk of exasperation, this is how the system works and how it avoids errors. Your job now is to lie back and picture yourself resting peacefully in the recovery room, hearing the doctor say that everything went great.

ANESTHESIA

One of the people asking you repetitive questions is the anesthesiologist or the nurse anesthetist. The former is a physician and the latter is, by training, a nurse. Both are highly qualified and will keep you safe and comfortable during the operation (your temporary best friend).

You may have had a chance before surgery to discuss whether to have a spinal or general anesthetic. (Epidural and spinal anesthesia are just variations on the theme and are discussed below.) Some doctors do arthroscopic surgery under **local anesthesia** (like at the dentist's office). If your doctor is experienced with this, or if you have some underlying medical problems, local anesthesia might be recommended. You often feel some pain with this type of anesthetic, so it is not usually the first choice. Thus, the majority of arthroscopies and all ligament and total knee surgeries are done under either spinal or general anesthesia.

Spinal or **epidural anesthesia** involves injecting some Novocain-type medicine into your back, which bathes the spinal cord and numbs you below the waist. This sounds scary, but I have never seen or heard of anyone *not* getting feeling back after a spinal. With this type of anesthesia, although you might feel an occasional vibration or pressure, *you will not feel any pain*. By having a spinal anesthetic, you can watch the arthroscopic portions of the operation on the TV monitors. Your brain has no idea it is your knee and it is just like looking at an aquarium (only without the bubbling guy in the dive suit).

General anesthesia, on the other hand, involves going to sleep with medicine injected through the intravenous (IV) line in your arm. Because your breathing center is anesthetized along with the rest of your body, the anesthetist will put some type of airway in your mouth and sometimes down your windpipe. Though you run the risk of a sore throat or some nausea, it is still a safe alternative for people who do not want to see or hear anything. Since the general anesthetic wears off more quickly than the spinal, it might allow you to leave the hospital sooner if you are having outpatient surgery.

THE OPERATING ROOM

The operating room (OR) looks just like it does in the movies. There are people bustling about in pajamas and others at tables in sterile gowns. (Everyone but the patient gets to wear a mask, but don't worry, you will still look festive in your own paper hat.) No matter how chaotic things look, the OR team is focused on getting you prepared for what is about to take place. All of their energies are centered on you. At one point, they will ask you to move from the gurney to the OR bed. Position yourself on the bed as instructed and do some *conscious breathing or imagery* of a wonderful, calm moment in your life.

There are tables covered with expensive instruments, many of which look like what you have in your garage: drills, screwdrivers, and the like. That's the great thing about orthopedic surgery—there's nothing slick or fancy. Simplicity is the rule. For example, the news media may report that someone had "cartilage repaired," but that is not what usually happens. If you have torn cartilage, 90 percent of the time we simply remove the damaged bits without affecting the remaining functional parts. Likewise, if you have a torn ligament, we make a new one. If you have a rough surface cartilage that cannot be smoothed or induced to heal, we cap it with some metal and plastic. What could be more bread and butter?

In Chapter 1, I compared arthroscopic knee surgery and open knee surgery. When using the arthroscope, the surgeon makes very small incisions ("portals" or "keyholes") in the skin into which to place the instruments. These incisions are so small many surgeons don't even close them with stitches—just some butterfly bandages. For ligament or knee replacement surgery, bigger incisions are made. These will be closed with stitches or staples that are removed in a week or two.

Ligament tears are reconstructed with either tendon pieces from another part of your body (autograft) or from a cadaver (allograft). Your doctor will discuss in some detail the pros and cons of each of these graft choices. Whichever graft is used, over time your body will grow blood vessels and nerves into it, making it your own.

With a total knee replacement, the knee never becomes "your own," necessitating some extra care of this knee for the rest of your life. In this operation, all of the rough, painful surface cartilage is cut away and replaced with metal and plastic pieces (like capping a tooth). The hard part in this operation is getting the pieces to stick to your bone. This is done with various combinations of cement, screws, and "bony in-growth" where the metallic surface is treated to encourage your bone to grow into it. No system is perfect, but by staying fit and caring for your knee, you should have a good, painless, functional joint for many years.

THE POST-OP RECOVERY ROOM

Once the surgery is over, the nurse in the recovery room will replace the anesthetist as your best friend. It is normal to be in some pain, but it is not normal to be in screaming agony. The nurse will ask you to gauge your pain, so be honest. The point here is to get you comfortable and as pain free as possible.

If you ever had a problem with pain medicine in the past (such as a high tolerance to pain meds, certain meds not working, or addiction problems), make sure you tell your doctor and anesthetist BEFORE the operation. The last thing you want is to make your recovery from surgery even harder because of pain management issues that could have been avoided with advance planning.

No matter what operation you have, from scope to ACL to TKR, health professionals want your knee to start acting like a knee right away. If you are in too much pain, you are not going to want to do the stretches and exercises that the nurses, therapists, and trainers ask you to do. For those of you who are wary of narcotics, refusing pain medicine is fine, as long as you are able to do the exercises, walk with crutches, and so on. In general, do not be afraid of moving about and doing your therapy after surgery, as it usually makes knees feel better—not worse. After all, your knee "wants" to be functioning like a knee as soon as possible.

With the stress of surgery in the rearview mirror, the next phase of the healthier you begins. Each day will bring you closer to a better knee. Be compulsive and deliberate, but do not be in a hurry. It might well be a year or so before you consider yourself back to normal. The key is to keep progressing in the right direction to a better knee and a healthier you. Healing can be encouraged but not rushed.

PART TWO

THE KNEE DOCTOR'S AFTER-SURGERY PROGRAM

THE CRITICAL
FIRST WEEK

Prong 2 of the Three-Pronged Attack:

Movement Patterns for Your Return

to Life

A WONDERFUL THING about any living creature, whether a person, puppy, or plant, is that it automatically attempts to heal itself after an injury. The problem is, left to its own devices, the knee does not necessarily continue to heal to the point where you can rip a slalom course, dunk a basketball, or sit comfortably on a plane to China. Those abilities require not just healing but also rehabilitation and training to return the knee to top condition.

The critical first week after surgery sets the tone for the coming weeks and months of recovery. This is where you must let your knee know, in a firm but gentle fashion, that you expect it to come back stronger and happier than it was before. In these post-op days, you must treat your knee like a child. It needs lots of guidance and encouragement. Most of all, it needs your attention, and that means your time.

Rather than being discouraged or depressed about all the things you cannot do right now, focus on what you can do and control—such as managing your pain, limiting swelling, hydrating, stretching, and strengthening. Sweat the small stuff. Not only does compulsiveness help your knee, it also keeps your brain occupied.

TAKE CARE OF YOUR INCISION

Keep the bandages, and thus the wounds, dry. In the first couple of days after surgery, drainage from the wound is normal. Sure, it's gross, but it's better to have the fluid come out of the knee than to stay in and slow your rehab. Most of the fluid is saline solution that was pumped into the knee during the surgery. With that in mind, make your bed with old but clean linens.

If the bandages get so wet and bloody that you can't stand looking at them, you may change them. First, thoroughly wash your hands. Pull down the stocking or Ace, remove the old gauze, and dab the wounds with some alcohol, witch hazel, or peroxide on a clean paper towel. Leave alone any tapes or pieces of gauze that are stuck. Re-dress with clean gauze bandages and replace the stocking or Ace. Remember, if using an Ace bandage, start from the toes and wrap evenly toward the knee. If you do not feel comfortable doing this, you can just leave everything alone until your next office visit.

For bathing, place an old stool in the shower stall or tub so you can sit for the first few weeks after surgery. Once you are cleared to shower, cover your knee in plastic wrap and afterward wipe down the wound with an alcohol-soaked paper towel. Most arthroscopy knees can get wet in the shower after two or three days, but they should not soak until the portals are completely healed, usually about a week. For ACL and TKR knees, wait until the stitches come out at seven to fourteen days before taking an unwrapped shower or bath. Another option is to take a shallow bath (six to eight inches deep) and keep your knees bent up, out of the water (which is also a good way to work on your flexion). Doctors have varying opinions on this, so always defer to your surgeon or nurse if there is any question.

MANAGE YOUR PAIN
MEDS WISELY

A prescription for a narcotic pain reliever will be given to you before your discharge from the hospital. Take enough of the narcotic to decrease pain so you can do your rehab and get some sleep, but not so much as to make you a zombie. **Driving a car or operating machinery is not allowed under any circumstances when taking such medicines.**

Try to fill your prescription beforehand so you do not have to stop on the way home from the hospital. Always take these medications with food and plenty of fluids (no alcohol!). If you experience an upset stomach or other undesirable side effects from the medicine prescribed, stop taking it and call your doctor. An alternative medicine may be suggested or you can stick to the over-the-counter protocol below.

Because narcotic medication can cause constipation and other problems (like making you sleepy and loopy), I encourage patients to switch to a program of over-the-counter pain medicines (naproxen, ibuprofen, or acetaminophen) one or two days after surgery. TKR patients, however, usually need narcotic medicines a bit longer. This over-the-counter protocol assumes you have normal-functioning kidneys and liver and no stomach problems. If there is any question, check with your doctor. You do not want to be in severe pain, but the sooner you can get off the narcotics, the better.

OTC PAIN MEDICINE PROTOCOL

Over-the-counter (OTC) anti-inflammatory alternatives that will give you the same dosages (400 mg of naproxen or 800 mg of ibuprofen) as a prescription medication:

- 2 naproxen (200 mg tablets) (e.g., Aleve) with breakfast
- 2 naproxen tablets with dinner

OR

- 3–4 ibuprofen (200 mg tablets) (e.g., Advil, Motrin, Nuprin) with breakfast
- 3–4 ibuprofen with lunch
- 3–4 ibuprofen with dinner

If your stomach cannot tolerate naproxen or ibuprofen, stick with acetaminophen for nonnarcotic pain relief:

- 2 extra-strength acetaminophen (e.g., Tylenol) three times a day (i.e., with meals)

Note: It is generally safe to combine naproxen or ibuprofen with your narcotic medication. You do not need to take acetaminophen (Tylenol) until you stop taking the narcotics, as most narcotics have some Tylenol in them.

Just as with the narcotics, if you have stomach upset or any other bothersome side effects from OTC medicines, discontinue use immediately. If you have previous ulcer or other gastrointestinal problems, stick to straight Tylenol. You should not take any other anti-inflammatory medicines at the same time as ibuprofen or naproxen. To build up the drug level to where it is most effective, try not to skip a dose. Usually by four or five days after surgery, you can stop taking all medicines except your vitamins. Consider taking a multivitamin with iron for one month after most surgeries and six months after a TKR. Although arthroscopy patients do not lose a huge amount of blood, replenishing your vitamin and mineral stores after the stress of surgery is rarely a bad idea.

Remember: Medications and vitamins are only supplements to the other post-op steps you are taking toward recovery, such as RICE, proper nutrition, and the three-pronged attack recovery program.

PRONG 2: MAINTAINING YOUR MOVEMENT PATTERNS

Movement patterns, which should begin right after surgery, are the second prong of my three-pronged attack on knee rehab (remember, the first prong is the exercise and stretching program). This is one of the main facets of my program that sets it apart: I do not want you to wait until you are "all better" to get back to your favorite activities. Re-creating some of the same movement patterns immediately after surgery that you made prior to surgery—whether they are gardening, loading a truck, playing second base, or dancing—will help keep your muscle memory alive, speeding recovery. From a surgeon who

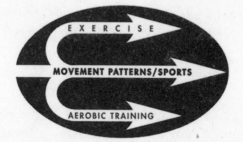

also happens to be a sports psychologist, I believe this is a vital aspect of a healthy mind-body approach to rehab.

Prong 3, aerobic training, will not start until at least a week or two post-op. Doing aerobic work such as cycling, treadmill, etc., is usually too much for the operative knee in week one. The repetitive nature of these motions can cause irritation and swelling. Hold off for now; I discuss aerobic training further in Chapter 7.

If you are an athlete, you need to perform sport-specific movement patterns that help re-create aspects of your sport. For example, if you are an avid tennis player, keep a racket nearby both as visual inspiration to stay on track with your post-op rehab and to literally practice your forehand and backhand. Your knee will better respond to the movement patterns if you give it a job it understands. Making *small, slow, deliberate* steps that mimic tennis footwork in the days after surgery will not harm your knee and will help retain your muscle memory. If the ceiling allows, you can even practice perfecting your serve. If you are a gardener, get potting soil for some indoor planting. Be creative. Remember, this is not just physical therapy but mental therapy as well. Basically, if something in the house does not get broken in this first week, you're just not trying. *Flip to Chapter 12 right now to get an idea of the movement patterns I want you to be doing very soon after your surgery and start thinking about how you might structure your own "Return to . . ." program.*

As for the pain, swelling, and other not-so-fun aspects of healing, the following tips will help you get through the critical first week. (At the end of the chapter there is a chart with activities for Day 1, Day 2, etc., following the operation, as well as a summary of the first week's goals.)

REDUCE SWELLING

Your first job after surgery is to get rid of the swelling you have and prevent any more from occurring. In arthroscopic procedures, much of the swelling is due to the saline that was pumped into the knee during surgery. With total knee replacement, the swelling is mostly a result of your knee being inflamed and angry from the bone cuts. From Chapter 2 you remember that swelling means it is time for more RICE.

Post-op RICE

R=REST. Large gains in rehabilitation are not going to be made by working harder at this stage (remember, you are working smarter, not harder). Your body has been through significant trauma from both surgery and anesthesia, and it needs to recuperate.

FITNESS = MOVEMENT + REST

You need to make a concerted effort in your rehab, but this must be accompanied by rest and recuperation. For example, when doing your stretches, *do your stretches,* don't just go through the motions. By making sure you are moving through your full range of motion and contracting your muscles completely, you are efficiently working your knee. This must now be accompanied by rest to allow those muscles to repair themselves before the next effort. This is why I recommend one day off a week from aggressive rehab work and a specific number of reps such as described in the sample workout in Chapter 3.

I=ICE. Use an ice bag or other icing device regularly. The goal in the first few days after surgery is ice 20 minutes every 2 hours. Repeat this throughout the day. Cold therapy helps reduce both pain and swelling. As described earlier in this chapter, after forty-eight hours you can usually change the dressing to a lighter layer of gauze held on by the stocking or Ace bandages. A lighter dressing allows the cold to get to the knee more easily. Again, if the wound gets wet, wipe it down with alcohol, witch hazel, or peroxide on a clean paper towel.

C=COMPRESSION (AND MASSAGE). The stockings or Ace bandages not only hold on the bandages but also help control swelling. Ideally, you should wear them for the first two weeks (unless it is the middle of the summer and you are really suffering). You can massage your knee comfortably right over the dressings, always stroking toward the heart (more specific massage instructions are discussed later in this chapter).

E=ELEVATION. It is essential to keep your leg elevated above your heart as much as possible to allow the excess fluid and blood to exit the knee. At least 15 minutes of every waking hour should combine elevation with passive extension (Chapter 2, ROM # 1). When sleeping, try to stay on your back with pillows elevating your leg. If you are a side sleeper, place a pillow between your knees with the surgery knee on top. Take some time to arrange yourself, as a good night's sleep is important for healing.

RECOVERING RANGE OF MOTION (ROM)

Week 1 Goal: Achieving Full Extension (Straightening) and Flexion (Bending) to 110 Degrees

Each day you will work steadily toward improving your range of motion. Here are some guidelines to follow.

CONTINUOUS PASSIVE MOTION (CPM) MACHINE

The CPM machine is used in many hospitals (and sometimes sent home with TKR patients) to elevate your leg while moving it through a designated range of motion. The leg is usually placed into the CPM soon after surgery, and the machine moves your knee from straight to as much bend as you can tolerate. Unfortunately, you will not get your knee entirely better by being passive. Knee rehabilitation is a predominantly active—not passive—process.

ROM Stretches

Once you leave the hospital, range of motion becomes your responsibility and one you need to take very seriously (see ROM stretches in Chapter 2). Again, the goal is full passive extension at least 15 minutes every hour in addition to the other ROM stretches. In most ligament surgeries, flexion (bending) tends to be easier to get back than extension (straightening), but it still needs attention. Conversely, patients who have had a TKR usually have to work a bit harder on flexion (bending) since their knees were often stiff for years before the surgery. Getting and maintaining full extension and 110 degrees of flexion may be uncomfortable, but it is crucial that you seek to achieve this in the first week.

Patella Mobilization

Mobilization (or massage) of the patella should be done at least 3 times a day for 5 minutes. In the beginning, massage right through the dressings. First, relax all of your leg muscles. Hold the patella (kneecap) between your thumb and forefinger and try moving it up and down as well as back and forth. Do this both with the leg fully straight and

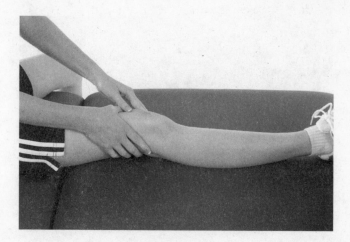

Patella mobilization

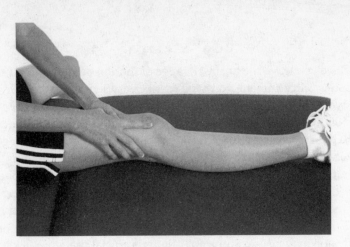

Patella mobilization

slightly bent. Once a lighter dressing is put on the knee, you will be able to feel your kneecap better. Patella massage is especially important after TKR and ACL surgeries where a patella tendon graft was used. Moving your patella shouldn't actually hurt, but might feel a bit strange at first.

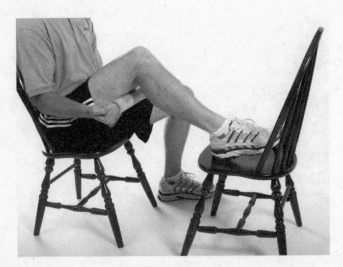

Muscle massage

MUSCLE MASSAGE

Massaging your muscles helps to reduce swelling, relieve soreness, and promote healing. With your foot propped up, massage from the toes all the way to the groin, in an effort to push the fluid toward your heart. Use a squeezing motion to mobilize swelling and a deeper, kneading-type stroke to relax the muscles of your leg and thigh. Do all four sides of your thigh: top (quads), bottom (hams), and sides. Spend extra time on any particularly sore areas, such as the hamstrings if your ACL graft was harvested from here.

You can massage your own legs, but having someone else massage them for you is obviously better. If you can't recruit anyone and your hands get tired, try moving your thigh over a foam roller or padded rolling pin (wrap a towel around it). (See photo page 88.) As with patella massage, you should massage your muscles at least 3 times a day in the first week. Hiring a massage therapist is a worthwhile investment, even if just to learn a few techniques that you can adopt at home.

REGAINING MUSCLE CONTROL

Though you feel a bit wobbly, muscle control will return with two key ingredients: deliberate practice and persistence. *It is best to start the ROM stretching from Chapter 2 and Level A exercises from Chapter 3 as soon as the anesthetic wears off.* Remember, don't just give the muscle a quick pull but slowly and deliberately contract the muscle, trying to recruit as many fibers as possible. One of the tricks used earlier to get your knee to understand what you want it to do was well-leg exercises (see Chapter 3). In other words, do the movement on the well leg first so your brain understands what you want to do on the operative leg. If any exercise causes significant pain, *stop* doing it until you check with your doctor, therapist, or trainer.

Nonathletes may get nervous the first time they feel some muscle soreness. Try to distinguish between muscle ache and knee pain—pain and swelling in the knee the day after you do something mean that you overdid it. Soreness or aching in your muscles the day after you do something means you are working hard to get stronger.

FOLLOW A SET SCHEDULE

Keeping a rehab routine in place gives you focus, and focused people tend to accomplish their goals in life. So if your goal is to get back in the swing of things, the next pages can literally help you chart your course.

Ultimately there is no difference in the way you rehabilitate from knee surgery and how an Olympic athlete rehabilitates. Furthermore, there is little difference in how an arthroscopy patient rehabilitates compared to an ACL reconstruction compared to a total knee replacement. Recovering from all three involves the same program, just on different time lines. More precisely, arthroscopy patients will probably follow the Level A exercise program for about a week post-op before moving on to another level of rehab work; ACL patients will do Level A for about two weeks; and TKR patients for at least three weeks. These are only ballpark figures since how soon you begin the next part of the program simply depends on how your knee is responding, not on any arbitrary schedule.

WEEK 1 SAMPLE POST-OP DAILY WORKOUT SCHEDULE

Day 1	
	• REST, REST, REST.
	• Keep your leg elevated.
	• Continue to hydrate.
	• Check your organization to ensure your space is comfortable and fun for the coming days.
ROM	• Passive extension, 15 min every hour.
	• Heel slides, 3 times a day or more.
	• Towel stretch.

EXERCISES	• Quad sets, 2 times a day or more. • Co-contractions, 2 times a day. • Leg raise with co-contraction, 2 times a day. • Ankle pumps: flex and extend your foot when your leg is elevated, 5 min every hour.
OTHER	• RICE at all times when not exercising. • Patella and muscle massage, 3 times a day. • Take medication on a regular schedule to stay ahead of the pain. • Touch-down crutch walking (keep this to a minimum!).

Day 2

	• REST, REST, REST. • Don't be afraid to move the leg! • Elevate when not moving. • Continue to hydrate. • Line up some good books to keep your brain exercising.
ROM	• Passive extension 15 min every hour. • Heel slides, 3 times a day. • Towel stretch.
EXERCISES	• Quad sets, 3 times a day. • Co-contractions, 3 times a day. • Leg raise with co-contraction, 3 times a day. • Ankle pumps, 5 min every hour.
OTHER	• RICE at all times when not exercising. • Patella and muscle massage, 3 times a day. • Take medication as needed. Decrease narcotics and begin over-the-counter protocol. • Change dressings as needed. • Touch-down crutch walking (again, keep to a minimum!).

(continued)

Day 3

	• Increase emphasis on range of motion. • Patience and good work, not necessarily *more* work. • Keep your leg elevated. • Put some good food in the system!
ROM	• Passive extension 15 min every hour. • Heel slides, 3 times a day. • Towel stretch. • Prone leg hangs, 2 times a day.
EXERCISES	• Quad sets, 3 times a day. • Hamstring sets, 3 times a day. • Co-contractions, 3 times a day. • Leg raise with co-contraction, 3 times a day.
OTHER	• RICE at all times when not exercising. • Patella and muscle massage, 3 times a day. • Medication—should now be using minimal narcotics. • Keep the dressing and wound dry. • Crutch walking—add more weight if no pain. (Keep walking to a minimum!) Use cat walk pose (p. 29). • Gentle movement patterns: Start moving your feet slowly and deliberately like learning a new dance move. • Don't forget well-leg and upper-body exercises.

Day 4

	• Motion, motion, motion! • Be confident that your knee can fully extend. • Make sure you are drinking fluids and eating well. • Keep your leg elevated when not exercising.

ROM	• Passive extension, 15 min every hour. • Prone hangs, 2 times a day. • Towel stretch. • Heel slides, 3 times a day. • Standing and seated flexion.
EXERCISES	• Quad sets, 3 times a day. • Hamstring sets, 3 times a day. • Co-contractions, 3 times a day. • Leg raise with co-contraction, 3 times a day.
OTHER	• RICE at all times when not exercising. • Patella and muscle massage, 3 times a day. • Medication: You should be off the narcotics at this point. Follow over-the-counter protocol. • Keep the wound dry and continue use of compression stockings. • Crutch walking: Slowly add more weight as you are ready. Get outside if weather is nice. Cat walk pose! Movement patterns!

Day 5

	• Enter "human" phase. • How often is the mental movie showing? • Motion! • If available, get on an indoor bike for well-leg motion and dumbbells for upper body.
ROM	• Passive extension 15 min every hour. • Heel slides, 3 times a day. • Towel stretch. • Standing and seated flexion.
EXERCISES	• All Level A exercises, but *do not* do exercises that cause pain.
OTHER	• RICE continues. • Patella and muscle massage, 3 times a day.

(continued)

- Medication: Follow over-the-counter protocol.
- Keep the wound dry and continue use of compression stockings.
- Crutch walking: Slowly add more weight. Keep your head up and facing forward. Cat walk pose.
- Hide the lamps and toss a ball around.

Days 6 and 7

- Prepare for first post-op visit with your physician.
- What your doctor will be looking for:
  - **reduced swelling**
  - **full extension**
  - **flexion to 110 degrees**
  - **strong quad set and co-contraction**
  - **patella mobility**
  - **smooth crutch or full weight-bearing gait**

ROM	• Do all ROM stretches now. • Passive extension, 15 min every hour. • Heel slides, 3 times a day. • Supine leg hangs, 3 times a day. • Cat walk pose. • Towel stretch. • Standing and seated flexion. • Standing extension.
EXERCISES	• All Level A exercises, except those that cause pain (mention these to your doctor).
OTHER	• RICE continues. • Patella and muscle massage, 3 times a day. • Medication: Start decreasing over-the-counter protocol. • Keep the wound dry and continue use of compression stockings.

- Movement patterns: Feet should start feeling happier.
- Crutch walking: Slowly add more weight. Keep your head up and facing forward. Cat walk pose.

Before your head starts spinning and you start thinking, "I can't do all of this," relax. Take a deep breath. First, remind yourself that although it seems overwhelming, once you get started, it all flows. Second, this is all going to make a difference, potentially for the rest of your life. Third, once you get in the routine it will be just that: routine. Slow and steady really does win the race, even when it comes to knee rehab.

So how does the Week 1 daily schedule you just read fit into your life? The following is what a day in your first one to three weeks after surgery might look like. Obviously this is an ideal schedule, but the closer you can get your life to look like this, the faster your knee will get better.

AFTER-SURGERY SAMPLE DAY

8:00 A.M.	Wake up, wash face, brush teeth. Cup of tea or coffee (decaf if you can stomach it). Warm-up: Upper-body, well-leg exercises, sit-ups: total 5–10 min. ROM stretches, slow: 10–15 min. Imagery or conscious breathing: 2 min.
9:00 A.M.	Light breakfast of fruit, oatmeal, watered-down juice. Put knee in passive extension position with ice bag while eating.
10:00 A.M.	1st exercise session (described above in the daily schedule).

(continued)

	Warm-up: 5 min.
	ROM stretches: 10 min.
	Level A exercises: 15–20 min
	Cool down with ROM stretches: 10 min.
	Ice: 5 min.
	Patella and muscle massage: 5 min.
	Ice: 20 min, passive extension while icing.
	Don't even try to find something interesting on TV at this time of the morning. Daydream until noon.
12:00 noon	Nap: 45 min.
	Wake up and repeat 8:00 A.M. warm-up routine, ROM stretches.
1:00 P.M.	Light lunch of sandwich on whole-grain bread, yogurt, and fluids.
2:00 P.M.	2nd exercise session: Same as 10:00 A.M. routine. Again, this will depend what day post-op you are and is described in the daily schedule above.
3:30 P.M.	Practice crutch walking or real walking.
	Movement patterns: swing a golf club or tennis racket, push a soccer ball, toss a football, etc.
5:00 P.M.	3rd exercise session: Remember, your exercise sessions will change subtly as the week progresses.

6:30 P.M.	Evening news (or *Brady Bunch* reruns).
7:00 P.M.	Healthy dinner.
	Family time.
8–10:00 P.M.	Massage, ice, ROM stretches. Make notes in your journal as to what might need more emphasis: Stretching? Exercise? Hydration? Rest? Don't include just physical needs, also think mental needs.
10:00 P.M.	Read an inspirational biography.
11:00 P.M.	Lights out.

OKAY, BUT WHAT'S NEXT?

As I've discussed, this book is designed to introduce the three-pronged attack of rehabilitation (exercises, movement patterns, and aerobic training) in a deliberate and quantitative fashion. Before introducing the next level of the attack, aerobic training, it's important to expand on your movement patterns.

REHAB= TRAINING= WORK= SPORTS

Training, work, sports, and now rehabilitation are part of your life. Such activities can almost always be quantified by matters of speed (how fast), volume (how much), and mental attitude. The good news is that you are almost finished with the boring part of your convalescence and can start adding activities that are both fun and useful for the rest of your life (adding up to FITNESS!). After knee surgery, I suspect that even getting back to work will be a pleasure.

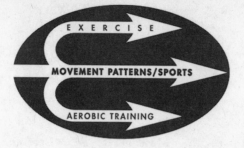

EXERCISE

MOVEMENT PATTERNS/SPORTS

AEROBIC TRAINING

Movement Patterns with Deliberate Practice

Every knee surgery patient is coming back to a sport, job, and lifestyle that is unique. Earlier in the book, I asked you to start practicing the movement patterns particular to that lifestyle so you do not completely lose the all-important muscle memory. Consequently, cyclists should get on a bike, ski racers should be weighting their downhill foot, drivers should move from the gas to the brakes, and factory workers should be stepping around a drill press, whether virtually (with imagery) or actually, as soon as possible. An important part of making yourself better after knee surgery is to practice these motions at a slow speed in a safe environment. Attempt to eliminate mistakes you made in the past. Tennis players: Are you bending your knees? Workers: Are you lifting with your legs? Basketball players: Are you facing the rim as you shoot? In the sport psychology world we call this "deliberate practice."

If you do something again and again with bad technique, you will never improve. Athletes with bad technique can usually find a coach or instructor to help them. Because most loggers and salesmen don't have coaches watching them, they need to act as their own coach. What's your position sitting in the car? Using the phone? Changing a tire? Can you be more efficient, stronger, and safer? (Of course you can!) Whether you're doing athletics or work, practice your movement patterns in a safe environment (good footing, no dogs knocking you over, etc.). Perform movement patterns slowly, methodically, correctly, *deliberately*.

Movement Patterns and Volume

Assuming you have established proper movement patterns at a safe speed, the next question is, how much? It seems almost too obvious to mention and yet this is where many people get into trouble. All patients, when returning from surgery, should be in "spring-training mode": limited volume. Nobody pitches nine innings during spring training. For example, after that first week post-op from your arthroscopy, if you cannot resist the urge to vacuum or pull some weeds, fine. Set your watch for fifteen minutes and when the alarm beeps, get back on the chaise longue for the rest of the hour. You can repeat this two or three times over the course of the day, but that should be it. Tomorrow you can do more, but the concept is to stay *below* the threshold of pain, not work right up to it. And I hope it goes without saying that on the first day back, you do not have to ski until dark or play three sets of tennis.

Adhering to such a schedule is easy at home; it is much tougher to maintain this limited activity level once you are back at work or with the team. These are some of the toughest decisions you, your doctor, trainer, and therapist must make. Try to establish some parameters with your boss or coach before getting back to your full-time, full-duty life. For example, return to your construction job on a Thursday so you have a weekend to recover after two days of work. Regarding sports, it's important to feel like part of the team. Rehabilitate in view of coaches and teammates but resist doing too much too soon. Your doctor will be more than happy to give you a return to work or sports note reflecting your limitations. Neither you nor your surgeon wants to risk a potentially successful result by being impatient.

UNDERSTANDING MUSCLES

Negative Talk, and Breaking
Through Roadblocks

MUSCLE QUALITIES

For the time being, put aside how you *think* you feel about exercise and look at an often ignored fact of nature: Your body loves moving. In a larger, philosophical sense, it does not matter whether you are the kind of person who says, "I hate exercise" or "I feel like I'm going crazy when I can't run my three miles a day." Your body yearns (okay, maybe quietly) to keep every muscle, every joint, every cell performing in the way it was designed. And it was designed to move.

To help you recover from knee surgery, my three-pronged program involves multiple muscle qualities. In addition to your biological mandate to move, knowing more about the qualities of those movements might help you understand why you should also *want* to move.

Balance

The center of gravity is the point of a body where it is pulled to Earth. Without your muscles, when your center of gravity lies outside of your base of support (e.g., your feet, your skates, or your skis), you'd fall over! Since we often spend time with our weight unevenly distributed, we use our muscles to keep us upright. The ease and grace that you see in athletes and dancers come from balance that is achieved with efficient muscular activity.

Balance, as with all muscle qualities, needs practice to improve. Balance is relatively easy to achieve on level ground with good footing, but it becomes more challenging with the addition of obstacles like ice, hills, and darkness. Water provides the safest environment for people who need to work on their balance (more on that in Chapter 9). Additionally, because of the buoyancy you experience in water, keeping your body centered to perform the exercises properly is no simple task. Obviously, all skills you learn in the water translate, with practice, to the land.

Motion (Flexibility)

In rehab circles, you hear references to needing range of motion before any other muscle qualities can be considered. Personally, I do not like to isolate one muscle quality from the others. However, if you lack full mobility, the joint will struggle to achieve balance, strength, coordination, etc. As a result, my program is designed to achieve a full range of motion while working on multiple muscle qualities.

Motion should be beautiful. Seeing someone struggle to get out of a car is a painful sight. You don't have to be Baryshnikov to achieve fluidity of motion. It is a quality you can develop with time and awareness. Flexibility refers to the elasticity of your muscles, ligaments, and tendons. As anyone with a stiff neck or tight hamstring will tell you, flexibility is key to allowing easy motion.

Flexibility and balance are two qualities commonly lost with aging. The decrease in flexibility is a physiologic process whereby our tissues lose water, making them drier, tighter, and more prone to injury. The only real fountain of youth is to keep moving.

Coordination

Coordination is the ability to perform complex movements smoothly without a loss of balance and with a minimum of muscle and brain activity. As you do more complicated and dynamic motions, you will test your coordination. In truth, a large amount of what we call coordination is simply muscle memory. The golfer sinking a million-dollar putt is relying more on muscle memory and less on his "thinking" brain to hit the ball. The golfer has hit such a shot hundreds of times, establishing a smooth highway between the spinal cord and muscle. When an adjustment in the movement is needed (e.g., a break in the putting green), coordination through muscle memory takes over.

Do not get discouraged when attempting unfamiliar motions—time is necessary to develop muscle memory (as the saying goes, one can never be too rich or too coordinated). A coordinated body moves with grace and—even better—less fatigue. Did you ever wonder why your friend beats you down the ski slope but never seems out of breath? That is because she is using her muscles in a coordinated, efficient manner and thus expending less energy.

Strength

Strength is the force a muscle can exert during a contraction. The amount of that force depends on the size of the muscle (the number of muscle fibers contracting) and the position of the muscle (if the muscle is working in an efficient range of motion). Strength may be the least isolated of all muscle qualities. If you are working on balance, coordination, and flexibility, the result is always some increase in strength.

Endurance

Endurance is the ability of the cardiorespiratory (heart and lungs) system to get oxygen into the blood and on to the muscles in order to perform long periods of work. Heart and lung capacity are rarely the limiting factors in recreational athletes because our muscles give out first. Muscular endurance is the ability of that muscle to perform repeated contractions over time with the given oxygen supply.

Not every athlete needs a great deal of endurance. An alpine skier is not terribly concerned with endurance but should be concentrating on strength and other qualities for the ninety-second plunge down the mountain. Some level of endurance, however, is needed by all of us, if only to avoid gasping for air midway up the stairs.

Speed and Quickness

Speed is perhaps the most magical of the muscle qualities on the athletic field. For those who have it, speed often masks deficits in the other qualities. Speed is the stardust that can turn a routine play into a score.

I encourage you to vary speeds in all aspects of your rehabilitation program. Not only will your speed improve, but speed changes will also improve balance and coordination, with quickness being another outcome. Quickness involves anticipation and, similar to coordination, is a muscle-brain response. As a result, quickness varies significantly with age and experience.

Breathing

In your preparation for surgery, you did some conscious breathing for relaxation (see Chapter 4), but you can also use breath control during physical activity. While cycling up that tough hill, concentrate on conscious breathing; feel how your body responds. During that knee rehab session, picture your breath filling your legs, stretching and relaxing your ligaments. As also mentioned earlier, exhale on the difficult phase of the exercise and inhale on the relaxation phase.

MY MUSCLE QUALITIES: A PERSONAL TRACKER

1 (poor, bad, nonexistent) . . . 5 (average, okay) . . . 10 (excellent)

Use the muscle qualities list below to rank yourself from 1 to10 according to some activities in your life. For example, you can test your balance by timing yourself on your single-leg stance or measure strength by the maximum number of reps for an exercise. Other examples are given below in the sample, but feel free to come up with your own. Revisit and revise this list to check progress and focus toward achieving your goals. Use the three-pronged attack: exercises, movement, and aerobic training in this book to improve your weak areas.

Balance: ___
Motion and flexibility: ___
Coordination: ___
Strength: ___
Endurance: ___
Speed and quickness: ___
Conscious breathing: ___

(continued)

Sample 1

Shane's self-evaluation: ACL reconstruction at two weeks post-op

Balance (single-leg stance): 3

Motion and flexibility (knee extension): 1

Coordination (quick step running): 5

Strength (bench press): 7

Endurance (crutch walking): 1

Speed and quickness (quick step running): 5

Conscious breathing: 9

Note: The same activity can evaluate more than one exercise quality.

Let's review Shane's self-evaluation at two weeks: A balance rating of 3 does not surprise me. What worries me most is Shane's lack of motion. As a result, I would have him go back to the ROM stretches, RICE more, get in the pool (see Chapter 9), and do no other activities for the next few days until his motion improves. Again, *nothing is as important postoperatively as range of motion.* He can use his proficiency at conscious breathing while working out his stiffness.

He used quick step running to assess his coordination as well as speed and quickness. This makes sense, since at two weeks post-op there are not many activities with these qualities he is allowed to do.

I think it is fine he used a bench press to check his strength. This would probably be measuring how his body responded to the stress of surgery rather than any true fitness at two weeks. Again, I would expect poor endurance until he goes farther in his aerobic training.

Sample 2

Fiona's self-evaluation: TKR at four weeks post-op

Balance (standing with eyes closed): 5

Motion and flexibility (knee bend): 7

Coordination (walking without limp): 7

Strength (quad extension 30°–0°): 5

Endurance (walking): 4

Speed and quickness (brake pedals): 3

Conscious breathing: 6

Fiona had a different operation from Shane, creating different emphases and different expectations at four weeks. Standing with eyes closed, even on both feet, is not so easy if one leg has a new knee. Bending a TKR tends to be tough, and Fiona is doing well. The strength and endurance will improve with time. Obviously if she is slow moving from the gas pedal to the brake (a key skill to practice!) Fiona might want to wait before driving herself.

Negative Talk

[When the going gets tough during your post-op recovery, keep in mind that you have a choice when it comes to mental attitude. Either you say things like, "I can do this" and "I'm getting stronger," or "I'll never get better" and "Woe is me." These last two phrases are examples of negative self-talk. Self-talk is the words and thoughts you use when describing yourself and can be either positive or negative, spoken or unspoken. In other words, the things you say to yourself and others affect not only your attitude but also your recovery.

Finding examples of negative talk is easy. The continuum of

injury plus surgery plus recovery is no fun, but getting down on yourself (or your coach, parents, kids, and so on) only makes things worse. You don't always say out loud what you fear inside, but even saying things to yourself can have a negative effect on your recovery. Negative talk can be self-defeating at a time when you need all the help you can get to propel yourself forward in a positive, healing direction.

That does not mean you minimize your concerns. Always ask questions and ensure you are taking the right turns on the road to recovery. Ask your doctor if something does not seem right: if the pain is increasing, if you spike a fever, if you seem to be losing motion, or if you have other indications that your knee is not recovering properly. These are physical issues, and as long as things are progressing, there is no need to be hard on yourself. Develop a habit of thinking and saying nice things about your knee and your progress. No one wants to be with a negative person—and that includes you! As I discussed in Chapter 3, start your day with some positive self-talk and carry that with you during your workouts.

Roadblocks to Recovery

Use this gift of extra time to ferret out anything and everything that works against optimal knee health. Things that work against your body's ability to move, perform, or, in this case, heal as perfectly as it can are considered barriers or roadblocks to performance. A common reason people work with sport psychologists is to develop techniques that allow them to blast through such roadblocks on the way to achieving their goals.

Here's one example: Rather than thinking about what you must *do* to achieve something, try to think about what you can eliminate to achieve it. (This concept should appeal to the couch potato in all of us.) Before the surgery, what were some roadblocks that kept you from playing or working as well as your talent might indicate? Consider the following:

- *Did you have unrealistic expectations?*
- *Does your living situation make it difficult to get out and exercise?*
- *Is there a lack of emotional or financial support in your life?*
- *Do you have too many commitments?*
- *Does your work help or hinder your knees' physical state?*

Additionally, for you athletes:

- *Are you experiencing pressure from your parents or coaches?*
- *Are you over- or undertraining?*

Over the course of the weeks and months that you have been dealing with your knee problem, you probably said a few things and made a few bargains with yourself: "After surgery, I'm going to eat smaller portions" or "When my knee is better, I'll get on the winner's podium." You can do these things, but not without breaking through the roadblocks that stopped you in the first place.

Not all roadblocks are self-imposed; you might be living with a number of external roadblocks to success.

- *Does your partner smoke, making it tougher for you to quit?*
- *Do you know how to prepare healthy foods so they taste good?*
- *Is your spouse a lazy slug?*
- *Is there someone at the office always bringing in leftover cake?*
- *Is your house so messy that you've given up ever getting organized?*

These questions might sound silly, but inertia is common to every one of us. This inertia—this state of doing nothing about a roadblock—affects our lives to the extent that we might avoid healthy change. Facing up to the inertia is step one in breaking through the roadblocks to good health for you and your knee.

I hope that the people in your life will respect this new you and will perhaps make healthy changes in their own lives. If not, it might be time for you to make some hard decisions. You cannot choose your relatives, but you can choose your job, your hobbies, your friends, where you live, what you eat, and more. Life is too short not to see a happy face smiling back at you from the mirror.

So go ahead, start treating your roadblocks like the dominoes they really are!]

AEROBIC TRAINING

Prong 3 of the Three-Pronged Attack

UP UNTIL NOW you have been working on various exercise qualities such as flexibility through ROM stretches, strength through exercises, and balance and coordination through movement patterns. The following aerobic-training programs provide more work on these qualities plus start to add an element of endurance, quickness, and speed. They are also keys to getting you back to your normal (or improved) life.

Endurance is the ability of the cardiorespiratory system to get oxygen to the muscles in order to perform long periods of work. Do not confuse endurance exercises simply with running (I already see the runners rolling their eyes). While running can build endurance, it is also hard on your knee cartilage, ligaments, and tendons. To mitigate this trauma,

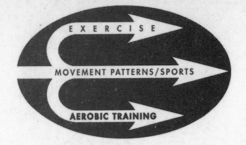

EXERCISE

MOVEMENT PATTERNS/SPORTS

AEROBIC TRAINING

most high-level runners use soft workouts, especially water running, as part of their training program. Cyclists, swimmers, and cross-country skiers are able to develop great endurance without pounding on their joints. For those of you who are superserious runners, knee surgery might be the impetus to get over your prejudices and consider supplementing your running with these softer workouts. Thus, the ideal aerobic-training program after surgery starts with walking and running in the water (see Chapter 9), and then follows the progression of cycling, the elliptical machine, the treadmill, and finally (if you *have* to) jogging and running outside.

I generally advise patients not to start aerobic training until one week after surgery, as it usually takes that long for even a knee arthroscopy to calm down. If you had anything more complicated than a "simple" arthroscopy, such as ACL or TKR, you probably shouldn't start these programs until two and three weeks post-op respectively. As always, check with your doctor.

These programs are to be done *in addition to* your other rehab. It will take planning to get organized, so you must become an expert at budgeting your time. Don't let distractions throw you off your game. The prime focus for the next couple of weeks is still your knee. Everything else can wait, your knee cannot. At the end of the chapter I summarize what your day/week should look like incorporating this aerobic training.

What follows are only examples. I recommend that you come up with your own aerobic-training schedule depending on the weather, the resources available to you, and your interests. Write down your program and go over it with your doctor, therapist, or trainer. Avoid pushing yourself harder or working out longer than your program calls for. Your fitness and endurance have taken a dive, but they will improve with time and persistence.

STATIONARY BIKE TRAINING PROGRAM

Use an exercise bike at the health club, home, hospital gym, or physical therapy facility; better yet, set up your own bike on an indoor trainer available at your local bike shop (see Resources). Put the bike in front of a TV to beat back the boredom.

The purpose of the bike initially is to increase blood flow and range of motion, not necessarily to work on your aerobic fitness or leg strength.

Getting Started

- Adjust the seat height so you are about an inch higher than your ideal cycling position. Your knee should be almost straight at the bottom of the pedal stroke. Ask a professional at the health club or bike shop to help you with your position. Not only will this improve your training efficiency, but it will add to your enjoyment and avoid aggravating other parts of your body.

- Slowly work the pedals forward and backward until you are confident you can make a full rotation without lifting your hip or standing up off the seat. You need about 115 degrees of knee flexion in order to ride smoothly.

- Your knee might be tight from swelling, so a little discomfort is normal and okay to work through. It should feel better as the session progresses. If cycling is causing significant pain, stop.

- Use minimal resistance initially. You want to focus on a smooth, circular pedal stroke.

- Once you are comfortable spinning on the bike, drop the seat height one inch and start the process over. You should now be in your proper cycling position with your knee bent to about 15 degrees at the bottom of the pedal stroke.

- Stretch and ice after each session.

LEVEL A

PURPOSE	Great range-of-motion stretch to help loosen up a stiff knee.
PROTOCOL	3 times a day: 5–10 min Can use as a warm-up prior to any workout
COMMENTS	• Promotes ROM after the first week post-op. • Forward and backward pedaling are recommended. • Take it slow, trying not to lift your hip off the seat. • Light resistance on the bike—only easy spinning!

After only one or two weeks post-op, this program may be easy for some, but your knee is not ready to crank hard on the pedals. At this point, you are using the bike just for motion and a change of pace. Later in your recovery you will concentrate more on technique, resistance, and endurance. Be sure you are comfortable with Level A before you begin Level B.

LEVEL B

PURPOSE	Light strength and endurance.
PROTOCOL	Light resistance: 5 min Medium resistance: 10 min Light resistance: 5 min **Total:** 20 min
COMMENTS	• Pedal speed: 80+ rpm (revolutions per min). • Keep the pedal speed the same during the 20 minutes. This means pushing a little harder during the 10 minutes of medium resistance.

- Make sure your bike adjustment is correct.
- Always stretch and massage the quadriceps and hamstrings after training.

LEVEL C

PURPOSE	Aerobic training when Level B is completely comfortable and easy.
PROTOCOL	Light resistance: 5 min Medium resistance: 10 min Heavier resistance: 5 min Medium resistance: 5 min Heavier resistance: 5 min Light resistance: 10 min **Total:** 40 min
COMMENTS	• "Heavier" resistance does not necessarily mean hard, just harder than "medium." When hard, you should still be able to turn the pedals at least 60 rpm. Your knee gets stronger by changing its workload. • Good stretch, ice, and massage afterward!

ELLIPTICAL MACHINE TRAINING PROGRAM

Elliptical machines and other run simulators offer a nice introduction to the real thing with less impact on the knee joint. Try it at a low speed and resistance to see if you like the feel. As with any machine, make sure you are instructed in how to use it before climbing on. After any of my workouts you should feel better, not worse.

- Speed: slow = very easy jog; medium = normal jogging pace
- Resistance: light = causes minimal fatigue; i.e., minimum increase in heart rate; medium = causes slight fatigue

LEVEL A

PURPOSE	Low-impact wake-up. Get the blood flowing. Introduction to jogging.
PROTOCOL	Slow speed/light resistance: 5 min Climb off for ROM stretching: 5 min Slow speed/light resistance: 5 min **Total:** 15 min
COMMENTS	• The elliptical machine is also a good place to warm up prior to any workout. • Maintain a nice upright posture! • Stretch and ice afterward.

LEVEL B

PURPOSE	Light strength, endurance, speed changes.
PROTOCOL	Slow speed/light resistance: 3 min Medium speed/light resistance: 3 min Repeat 2 more times **Total:** 18 min
COMMENTS	• An intro to endurance training while increasing the speed of movement. • The point is not to get a big muscle burn, but rather to tolerate the knee moving faster. • Stretch well after the workout!

LEVEL C

PURPOSE	Aerobic training when Level B is completely comfortable and easy.
PROTOCOL	Slow speed/light resistance: 5 min Medium speed/light resistance: 5 min Fast speed/light resistance: 5 min Medium speed/medium resistance: 5 min

Fast speed/medium resistance: 5 min

Slow speed/light resistance: 5 min

Total: 30 min

COMMENTS
- "Fast" speed might not be fast; it is just faster than "medium." Changing speeds is the key, not your actual speed.
- Proper cooldown is now part of your life.

TREADMILL WALKING PROGRAM

Walking on a treadmill can begin as early as one week post-op for arthroscopies, two weeks post-op for ACLs, and three weeks post-op for TKRs. As always, check with your doctor or therapist for a time line that suits your situation.

A treadmill allows you to adjust the speed and incline of the surface. Thus in this controlled environment, you can retrain your muscles to smooth out your gait. For example, this is the time to practice pointing your feet in the direction you're walking—not the Charlie Chaplin thing you've gotten into the habit of with your sore knee. In the process, you gain balance, coordination, and strength. Finally, the treadmill can help you build endurance as you increase the intensity of your program. As always, make sure you are familiar with how your particular machine works.

Increase your strength initially by walking uphill rather than speed walking. Similarly, begin a jog progression (see Return to Running in Chapter 12) with a slight incline to decrease the stress on your knee that comes with flat or downhill running. Be patient, and you will be running outside pain free in due time!

- Speed: slow = 2–3.5 mph; medium = 4–5.5 mph; fast = 6.0+ mph
- Incline: flat = 0%; low = 3–5%; medium = 5.5–10%; high = 10.5–15%

LEVEL A

PURPOSE	Improve gait, balance, and coordination.
PROTOCOL	Slow speed/flat: 5 min Break for ROM stretching: 5 min Slow speed/flat: 5 min **Total:** 15 min
COMMENTS	• Work on a smooth gait in this controlled environment. • Maintain an upright posture—think "five-star general."

LEVEL B

PURPOSE	Light strength and endurance. Regain your sanity.
PROTOCOL	Medium speed/low incline: 3 min Medium speed/medium incline: 3 min Repeat 2 more times: **Total:** 18 min
COMMENTS	• The incline will strengthen your leg and thigh muscles. • No limping allowed! • Swing arms to assume a normal gait. • Stretch calf, quads, and hams well after workout.

LEVEL C

PURPOSE	Aerobic training when Level B is comfortable and easy. You are still walking!
PROTOCOL	Medium speed/low incline: 5 min Medium speed/medium incline: 5 min Fast speed/low incline: 5 min Fast speed/medium incline: 5 min Fast speed/low incline: 5 min

Medium speed/low incline: 5 min
Total: 30 min

COMMENTS
- "Medium" and "fast" have been ballparked above, but don't hesitate to make some adjustments. The important thing is to change speeds and feel smooth.
- The Return to Running program in Chapter 12 assumes you have completed a program similar to this first.
- Proper cooldown—always!

SNOWSHOE TRAINING PROGRAM

Snowshoeing is a fun activity that you can usually begin safely two weeks post-op for arthroscopies but closer to four weeks for ACLs and two months for TKRs. No matter when you start, stay on relatively flat terrain for about a month before trekking gentle slopes and hills.

- Snowshoeing is a great winter activity for aerobic conditioning, strength training, and enhancing balance and coordination. Plus, it gets you outside breathing some fresh air.
- During the first few months post-op, stick to the trails you know. This is not the time for a backcountry adventure.
- Use ski poles to assist balance and to provide a smooth gait.
- You should have a normal gait on dry ground, no swelling, and excellent range of motion before snowshoe training.
- Your initial flat terrain experience should be no longer than 20 minutes.
- Gear: Don't carry a heavy backpack, but bring along water or an energy drink. Bring your cell phone in case you fall. And try to bring a dog—yours or borrow a neighbor's—for someone to talk to. Maybe leave the iPod home, enjoy the quiet, and listen to your breathing.

- Stop every 10 minutes or so to drink some water, stretch, and pat the dog.
- Increase your exercise time gradually.

LEVEL A

PURPOSE	Light endurance, strength, balance, and coordination
PROTOCOL	Flat terrain: 20 min
COMMENTS	• Use ski poles. • Bring water for you and the dog. • Stretch well after the workout.

LEVEL B

PURPOSE	Light to moderate endurance and fresh air.
PROTOCOL	Flat terrain: 30–50 min
COMMENTS	• Keep using ski poles. • Don't let the dog step on the back of your snowshoes! • Remember to cool down and stretch.

LEVEL C

PURPOSE	Aerobic training when Level B is too easy.
PROTOCOL	Interesting terrain, but still free of significant obstacles such as roots, logs, etc: 60–90 min
COMMENTS	• Poles are now optional. • Feel good co-contractions of your thigh muscles, especially when going up and down hills. • Have fun! How great is it to breathe some cold air?

AEROBIC TRAINING SAMPLE DAY

The following is what an "ideal day" (at least for your knee) might look like at this point in your rehab. Remember, you're trying to balance just the right amount of stress for your knee with the right amount of rest. This is ballpark timing:

- Arthroscopy: one week post-op
- ACL: two weeks post-op
- TKR: three weeks post-op

8:00 A.M.   Wake up!
Warm-up: Sit-ups, upper body, or well leg: total 5–10 min.
ROM stretches—slow, concentrate!
In the shower, replace singing with positive self-talk.

9:00 A.M.   Light breakfast of fruit, oatmeal, watered-down juice.
Put knee in passive extension position with ice and saddlebag/purse while eating.

10:00 A.M.   1st exercise session:
Warm-up: Level A stationary bike, or elliptical machine.
ROM stretches: 10 min.
Level A exercises: 15–20 min.
Cool down with ROM stretches for 10 min and then 5 min on the stationary bike or elliptical.
Simple movement patterns with Imagery (virtual skiing, tennis, baseball, etc.): 10 min.

(continued)

Patella and muscle massage: 5 min.

Ice: 20 min, passive extension and heel slides while icing.

Topic for thought until noon: *How can I simplify my life?*

12:00 noon   Nap: 45 min.

Wake up and repeat 8:00 A.M. warm-up routine, ROM stretches.

1:00 P.M.   Light lunch of sandwich fixings on whole-grain bread, yogurt, and fluids.

2:00 P.M.   Attend to work, family issues such as bills, etc. Put your knee in either a straight or flexed position so you will be getting some rehab done at the same time. While you're on the phone, try the cat walk pose to get full extension. When you're bored with that, do some single-leg balances.

3:30 P.M.   Clean up around the house as part of your movement patterns (ultimate multitasking!).

4:00 P.M.   2nd exercise session: You should be warmed up from the housework. Now give yourself a good stretch. Do your next exercise session similar to the morning's, but at least two days a week get in the pool for a water workout.

7:00 P.M.   Healthy dinner.

8–10:00 P.M.   Massage, ice, ROM stretches. Watch a ball game and see yourself on the field. Move with confidence.

10:00 P.M.	**Read something by an author you've never heard of.**
11:00 P.M.	**Lights out.**

RETURN TO NORMAL ACTIVITIES

Try to set a strict return-to-work schedule with your boss so you do not overdo things when getting back on the job. (Your boss might be worried about you not working hard enough—I am worried about you working *too* hard.) If you do not put limits on yourself, you wind up working until it hurts and thus set back your rehab. Do the same with your Return to Sports (Chapter 12). Plan times in the workday to ice and elevate (bring some in a cooler). You can do it, it just takes planning.

At any point, if your knee feels great after doing something, resist the urge to do more. On the other hand, if your knee is sending you distress signals about an exercise or activity, stop, RICE, and avoid that movement until you can discuss it with your doctor or therapist.

There is no crystal ball for the return to full activities. Many factors are involved, including biology (the healing time), the conditioning of the rest of your body, and your mental preparedness. When you return to activities is a decision for you, your doctor, your therapist, your athletic trainer, as well as your employer, coach, and family. Ultimately, though, the knee makes the final decision.

TESTING THE WATERS

The Ultimate Soft Workout

NO MATTER WHAT type of knee surgery you had, chances are good that your doctor may recommend a course of aquatic or water therapy. Here's why:

- Water is the ultimate soft workout.
- Water greatly facilitates joint movement as rough cartilage surfaces separate by "natural traction" to allow motion with less pain.
- Being in water allows your muscles to move, stretch, and work without the stress of gravity.
- Since your knee is not in pain in the water, you can get a great workout for all muscle groups.

Despite the fact that land is where we spend the majority of our lives, our existence began in an aquatic environment and the physical and mental benefits of that environment remain very real. We northern knee surgeons are jealous of our colleagues in the South where pools and aquatic classes for rehab are more widely available. Water exercise is not an imperative, but it certainly feels good. I made a promise to you in the Introduction to give you only activities that would make your knee better without wasting your time. Water therapy is one of those activities.

After your sutures have been removed and the wounds have healed—usually by two weeks post-op—it's safe to begin water therapy. You can get into the water before this by covering the wounds with waterproof dressings or plastic bags, but this technology is less than perfect. To be safe, ask your surgeon before submerging your knee in any water.

When you perform most weight room exercises, your muscles are not actually working through a full range of motion. When you lift your leg against gravity, the weights will provide resistance. But when you lower your leg back to the starting position, there is no resistance and you can coast. In the pool, on the other hand, the water provides resistance—in all directions! I call water exercises "isophysiologic" since they present your muscles with uniform resistance through the entire arc of motion. In water you can strengthen muscles with minimal risk of tearing or injury. Strengthening through the full range of motion also ensures that flexibility is not sacrificed for strength improvement. The relaxation effect of water, combined with the decrease in gravity, allows opposing muscle groups to relax and thereby gain flexibility.

To enhance your water training program, get some type of flotation device such as a vest, foam noodle, belt, or barbells, which will allow you to perform certain exercises more efficiently. This equipment, available at many sporting goods stores, will be a worthwhile investment since after rehabilitating your knee, you (or the kids) can continue to use it for years to come (see Resources). Soft workouts such as water sessions are a terrific way to burn calories and keep out constantly beating up your joints.

Break down any roadblocks you have to water therapy. Find a gym, health club, rehab facility, or even a nearby hotel with a pool. In fact, even if you do not do the exercises, just getting in the pool and moving about gives enormous benefits. The bigger the surgery, the more important it is to avail yourself of the soothing effects of water. Not being able to swim is no excuse: Try these exercises in chest-high water. If you can swim, start off in water over your head so that you are not standing directly on the pool floor (to eliminate as much gravity as possible). Just fifteen minutes in the water two or three times a week over the first two months post-op will significantly enhance your recovery. That's guaranteed. While a visit to the steam room or sauna is tempting, avoid these in the first month or so post-op. Not only can these rooms be slippery, but they are dehydrating. If you had more than a simple knee scope, you probably have not yet replaced your surgical blood loss.

Following are five basic water exercises along with workout tables according to your recovery level. Try doing the exercises for a set number of minutes rather than number of repetitions. This is a good way to avoid rushing any motion. Concentrate on practicing each motion deliberately and let yourself be a kid!

WATER TRAINING PROGRAM

DEEP-WATER WALKING AND JOGGING
FORWARD/BACKWARD

Purpose: Ideally, doctors would have everyone walking and jogging in the water before attempting these activities on land. This way you practice these basic movement patterns in a safe, forgiving environment.

Starting position: Stand vertically in deep water with a flotation device.

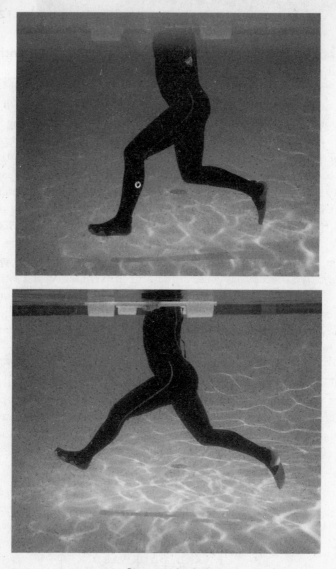

Deep-water jogging

Action: Start with some easy "walking" both forward and backward. The deep water eliminates gravity, and your knee loves it. Once you feel you are water walking smoothly in the deep end, shift into an area with neck-deep water. Proceed to the shallower areas as you get stronger. Pretend you are in finishing school, with a tall, upright position. Glide!

In addition to countering the effects of gravity, water provides resistance for muscle strengthening. Once you're walking well in the pool, head back to the deep end and start jogging. Before you know it, you'll be running up a mountain!

Note: Remember to do everything forward and backward, starting with slow, deliberate motions. The variations of the walking/running theme are endless, so feel free to make up games for yourself, such as interval "sprints" (speed changes).

LEG LIFTS

Purpose: This is a great core-strengthening exercise, again with endless variations.

Starting position: Using your flotation device, stand upright in deep water.

Action: Maintaining an upright posture, raise your legs to a 90-degree angle with your torso, or as high as possible. Feel the strength in your back and abdomen.

Note: The water is a great place to work on core exercises since the buoyancy is constantly pushing you to the surface and challenging your position.

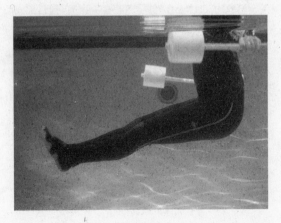

Leg lift

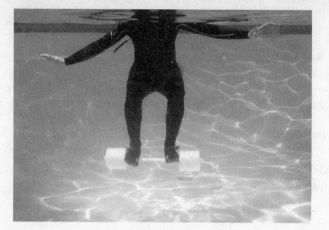

Barbell squat

FLUTTER BOARD OR BARBELL SQUATS

Purpose: Improve balance and motion.

Starting position: Stand with both feet on a heavy flutter board or barbell in deep water.

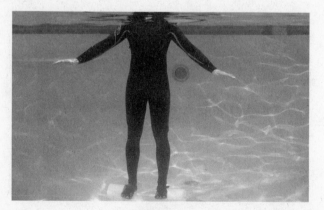

Barbell squat

Action: Allow the board to rise while you slowly flex your knees. Then press the board toward the pool bottom.

Challenge: Increase your speed.

SKIING

Purpose: A fun, dynamic exercise to work on lateral motion, speed and quickness.

Starting position: Using your flotation device, stand upright in deep water.

Action: Bring both knees up toward your chest and push them down at a 45-degree angle to the right, bring your knees back to your chest, and push them down 45 degrees to the left. Think moguls!

This is also a great exercise for your abdominal muscles. Feel the strength in these core muscles to increases the efficiency of the exercise.

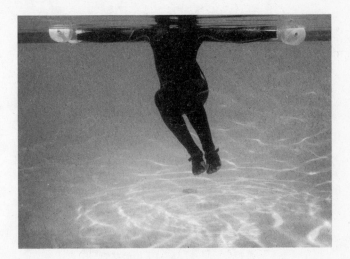

Skiing

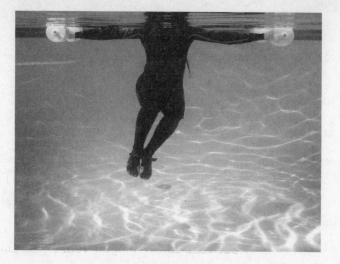

Skiing

Note: Arthroscopy patients can move to chest-deep water, pushing off the pool floor, as soon as they feel good. ACL and TKR patients should probably wait until six weeks post-op.

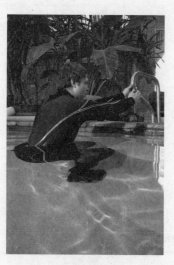

Ladder squat

LADDER SQUATS

Purpose: To improve knee range of motion.

Starting position: Stand on the bottom rung of the pool ladder or stairs and hold the hand bar without using a flotation device.

Action: Squat into the water to stretch and work on ROM at your knee. The water takes the weight off so you can safely and comfortably squat lower than on land.

Sample Water Workouts

I do not like to put time constraints on your knee, but it might help to have some ballpark guidelines:

Arthroscopy	Level A: 1 week post-op (or as soon as wounds are dry) Level B: 3 weeks post-op Level C: 6 weeks post-op
ACL reconstruction	Level A: 2 weeks post-op (or as soon as stitches are out and wounds are dry) Level B: 4 weeks post-op Level C: 8 weeks post-op
TKR	Level A: 2 weeks post-op Level B: 6 weeks post-op Level C: 8 weeks post-op

LEVEL A

PURPOSE	Flexibility, balance, and feeling better in general.
PROTOCOL	Deep-water walk: 5–10 min Leg lifts: 1 min Barbell squats: 2 min

(continued)

Deep-water walk 5 min
Ladder squats: 2 min
Total: 15–20 min

COMMENTS
- Promotes greater range of motion after the wounds are closed and dry.
- These can be done twice a day if you have easy access to a pool.
- Go slow and steady—*deliberate practice!*
- Excellent session for working out stiffness in the morning or at the end of the day.

LEVEL B

PURPOSE   Light strength, endurance, and speed.

PROTOCOL
Forward jogging: 5 min
Leg lifts: 1 min
Backward jogging: 5 min
Skiing: 2 min
Barbell squats: 1 min
Forward jogging: 5 min
Ladder squats: 1 min
Total: 20 min

COMMENTS
- Begin changing the speed of your movements in the water (e.g., 1 min slow, 1 min fast, 1 min slow, etc.).
- You can move from one exercise to the next without rest to get a bigger aerobic workout.
- Always finish with a stretching session.

LEVEL C

PURPOSE   Strength, endurance, and fun training.

PROTOCOL
Forward jogging: 5 min
Forward running: 5 min

Backward jogging: 5 min
Backward running: 2 min
Swim 2–4 pool lengths
Forward jogging: 3 min
Forward running: 5 min
Forward jogging: 5 min
Total: 30 min upright plus swim

COMMENTS
- Backward running is really tough. Do it for 2 minutes at a slightly higher speed than a jog.

- Use a crawl, side, or backstroke on your swim. Feel the leg motion at your *hips*, not your knees!

- Running is not sprinting. You cannot sprint for 5-minute intervals, but you could throw in some 15-second sprints along the way.

I have nothing against lap swimming so long as you do that in addition to "vertical" water exercises. Stick to the strokes mentioned above and really focus on the motion at your hips, feeling strength coming from there and the rest of your core muscles. Caution to ACLs and TKRs: no breast-stroke kick (otherwise called a frog kick) for six months post-op. Also, the biggest danger when doing water exercises is the pool deck! Be careful getting in and out.

PRONG 1, LEVEL B

Four New Exercises and Noise Reduction

LEVEL B EXERCISES are the next step up from your ROM and Level A exercises. You may begin these as early as two to three weeks post-op and continue until you have them mastered and are ready to move on to Level C (Chapter 11). As always, I want to keep the time frame vague to allow you to progress through the program *at your knee's pace.* You should not feel held back or, for that matter, pressured to advance. Again, no two knees are the same and will not respond identically to the "same" operation (since there is no such thing!).

For those of you who had "simple" arthroscopic surgery, Level B can start happening anytime after the critical first week. (Again, I say "simple" meaning that no big incisions

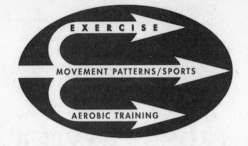

were made, understanding there is nothing particularly simple about it.) ACL reconstruction patients should be thinking about Level B around two weeks after surgery and TKRs from about four to six weeks post-op. Each new move is designed to rehabilitate your knee and minimize pain, not serve as an end in itself.

Here are some rules of thumb regarding readiness: Moving on to Level B assumes you are doing pretty well and perhaps feeling a bit bored with Level A. You might not be able to perform all of the Level B exercises perfectly, but do the ones you can. With a bit more healing time, and *deliberate practice,* you will soon be doing them all with excellent form. Use one of the aerobic training programs (stationary cycling, treadmill, or elliptical) or core exercises (e.g., sit-ups) to get a good warm-up. Always end with stretching and a cooldown activity (same as your warm-up or—better yet—water exercises). Be sure to exercise *both* legs, but do a few extra reps on the surgical leg to help get your body back in balance.

If you have had bilateral knee replacements, I suspect you have already discovered that one knee is a bit better than the other. Your knees, like the rest of you, are not perfectly symmetric. With bilateral TKRs, it may be longer before you are ready to shift into Level B, as you can proceed only as quickly as your worse knee.

One muscle quality that is left out of many recovery programs is *speed*. You should have started working on changing speed during your exercises, movement patterns, aerobic training, and water exercises. It won't seem like you are moving fast, because you aren't. You certainly will not be moving at work pace or sports competition pace, but it is the *change* in speed that you are looking for—even if it is slow, slower, and slowest! The changes in speed prime your neuromuscular system for life challenges to come.

LEVEL B EXERCISES

These four exercises are merely variations on Level A— and that is exactly the point. They build on what you and your knee already know. Combined with your movement patterns and aerobic training programs, these moves are all your knee needs and, frankly, all it can handle at this point.

DOUBLE-LEG SQUATS
(WITH OR WITHOUT STABILITY BALL)

Purpose: To improve functional strength and balance.

Starting position: Begin with your feet shoulder-width apart. Hold a chair or other secure object as in Level A, or, if

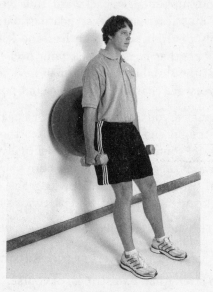

Double-leg squat

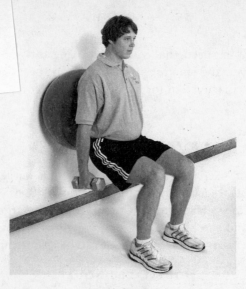

Double-leg squat

you're feeling good, add the stability ball (aka physioball, exercise ball) and/or dumbbells (as pictured). This adds a new element of balance—and challenge. Place your feet just in front of your hips and lean backward, thus working slightly different muscles than the standard squat. Keep your weight evenly distributed on both legs and keep your feet flat on the floor (that is, don't raise your heels). Depending on the size of the stability ball, you may have to move your feet farther forward than your normal squat position.

Action: Squat as if you are sitting down in a chair. Keep your lower back straight and strong. And tighten those abs! Start by doing quarter squats to 45 degrees; eventually, you may go down as low as 90 degrees. You are not born knowing how to squat properly, so have someone knowledgeable critique your technique. Do at least 3 sets of 10 reps, twice a day.

Challenge: Heavier dumbbells.

DOUBLE-LEG HAMSTRING BRIDGES

Purpose: To strengthen hamstrings, of course.

No one has strong enough hamstrings. No one. Most people

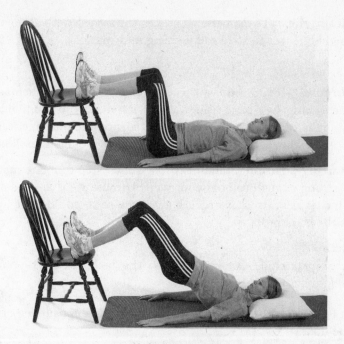

Double-leg hamstring bridge

stretch their hamstrings and strengthen their quads, but not enough people do the opposite. The hamstrings are a friend of the ACL, so whether you're recovering from an ACL tear or you'd like to avoid one, get those hamstrings pumped.

Starting position: Lie on your back with your heels on a chair or bench. Your hips and knees should be flexed to 90 degrees, with your arms out to the side for stability. The chair should be on a rug; otherwise you'll shove it across the room.

Action: Press your heels into the chair and lift your hips until they are well off the floor. Lower your hips without touching them to the floor, and repeat. Strive for 3 sets of 10 reps, twice a day.

The key to this exercise is to press your heels into the chair. You can put your feet on a stability ball rather than a chair, and the rolling will allow more motion in your knee.

Ideally, the ball's diameter should be the same length as your thighbone (see Resources for sizing information).

LATERAL STEP-UP

Purpose: Moving sideways is part of everyday life, such as negotiating wet or icy sidewalks. Lateral step-ups combine strength, coordination (agility), and balance into one practical motion. They work your knee and your outer thigh muscles.

Starting position: Stand next to a 3-inch step or a box that is strong enough to hold your weight (most steps are about 7 inches tall). As your strength increases, so should the height of the box/step.

Action:

1. Step laterally (sideways) onto the box and shift your weight completely to that leg.

2. Push down into the box while lifting the opposite leg off the floor.

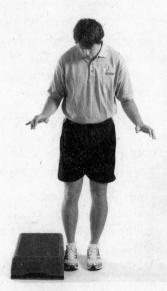

Lateral step-up

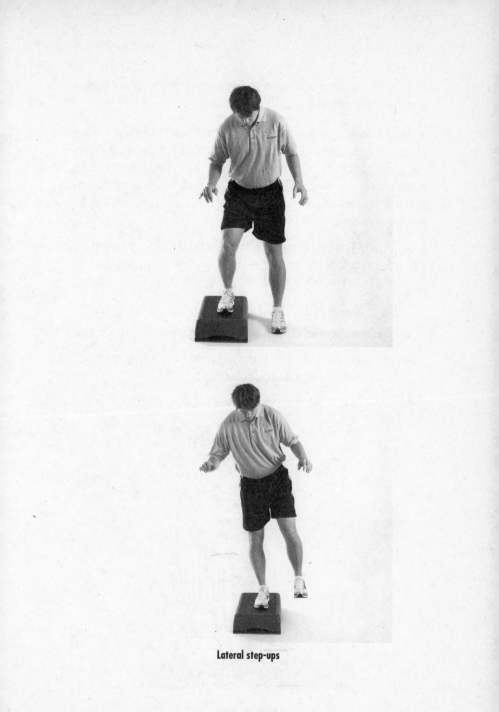

Lateral step-ups

3. Stand up fully without locking your knee. Maintain a good co-contraction.

4. Slowly lower your nonstanding foot back to the floor. This is sometimes called the "eccentric" part of the exercise (lowering the weight). Eccentric motions are often better than "concentric" motions (lifting the weight) when it comes to gaining strength. Return to starting position. Do 2 sets of 15 reps, twice a day. Go slow!

Challenge: The key is *not* to push off the floor but to push on the stepping foot. Keep the weight on this stepping foot as you slowly lower yourself down.

SINGLE-LEG SQUATS

Purpose: To become strong and balanced, one leg at a time.

Starting position: Stand with your weight on your front leg, using a chair or table for balance.

Action: Perform strong, slow, even squats. Start by going

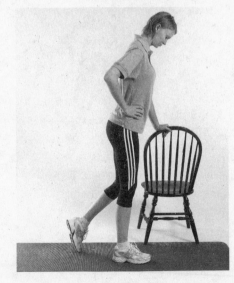

Single-leg squat

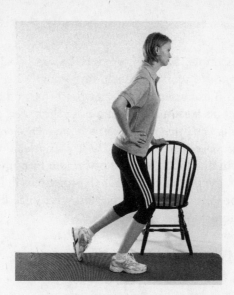

Single-leg squat

down only about 30 degrees (barely bending your knee). Slowly progress deeper as you get stronger. Lift your back leg and lose the chair as your balance improves. This is a tough exercise: 3 sets of 6 slow reps, twice a day.

The squat is such an important motion in life that I put variations of it in all three exercise levels. Single-leg squats, like leg balances, should be done obsessively. That means when you are in line at the DMV, at the grocery checkout, or on hold with your HMO, you should do some single-leg squats.

FITTING LEVEL B
INTO YOUR LIFE

All four of these exercises are vital motions for your knee's health. Along with your exercises and movement patterns, add different aerobic training programs over the course of the week depending on your choice or the weather (see Chapter 8). Structure your week into hard days and easy days. For example, Monday, Wednesday, and Friday can be 60- to 90-minute workouts including your ROM stretches, Level A and B exercises, movement patterns, and an aerobic activity such as treadmill walking or cycling. *Feel free to look ahead to Chapter 12 and start incorporating some more advanced sport-specific movement patterns.* These activities do not have to be done in one block but can be broken into multiple sessions. Only if you stick to this rehab program will I be able to fulfill my promise of getting you and your knee better than before the injury or surgery.

Background Noise

My job is to help get your knee feeling better. I try to eliminate anything that gets in the way of this. I appreciate that your days are already crowded with work, family, hobbies, and myriad other activities. With such busy lives, the concept of knee surgery combined with a lengthy rehabilitation program is difficult to imagine. I hope you are making the best of your recovery process by using the time to put things in focus and making positive changes in your life. You started those changes in your pantry and refrigerator by getting rid of the junk food. Now I'd like you to go through the rest of the house with that same purge mentality.

Often what keeps us from accomplishing more in life and consequently enjoying things more is what I consider "background noise." Background noise is all the stuff that is going on around you that tends to be unimportant and yet is a distraction. Background noise is having so much junk cluttering a room that you spend an hour looking for your car keys. Background noise is misplacing pieces of the bike rack so next summer, when you want to bring bicycles on your vacation, you wind up buying a new one. To make matters worse, you never throw the old one away, therefore adding to the clutter! Background noise is having the kids in so many activities that you never have time for yourself and thus wind up fat, cranky, and not even enjoying your child's company.

Try this: Spend fifteen minutes in the messiest room in your house. Put things back where they belong (you are performing movement patterns!) and, for Pete's sake, throw some things away! Now sit down to stretch and ice your knee, and observe what you've just accomplished. Impressive, right? And that's what you accomplished in just fifteen minutes. Getting rid of the background noise makes it easier to hear the fun and important things that are going on in your life.]

SAMPLE WEEKLY WORKOUT/ SAMPLE DAY

The following is a sample weekly workout table and a schedule of how these workouts might fit into an "ideal day," where taking care of your knee is the main emphasis. They are similar to ones in Chapter 6 but now include some of the new exercises and other elements I have since discussed. Note that the workouts are divided into hard and

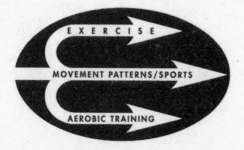

easy days. The hard days contain all elements of the three-pronged attack: exercises, movement patterns/sports, and aerobic training.

Remember: these are just suggestions. If you're a professional athlete or a retiree, you obviously have more time to work through the programs. If you are a businessperson who is going back to work soon after surgery, getting in a workout routine is more of an effort but an effort you must make or—trust me—you will still be struggling six months down the road.

Time is not as important as consistency. I do not expect all of you to find three hours a day to dedicate to your knee, but I do expect you to spend *some* time each day. I absolutely expect you to make your knee rehab part of your everyday activities. If you are not embarrassed at least once by someone catching you doing your squats on the elevator, you are not doing enough!

One last bit of business: Smile and have fun—you're getting better!

LEVEL B SAMPLE WEEKLY WORKOUT SCHEDULE

DAY	EXERCISE	TRAINING	MOVEMENT PATTERNS
Monday (hard)	*Morning* • ROM stretches • Level A exercises *Evening* • ROM stretches • Level B exercises	*Choose one* • Elliptical *or* • Cycling *or* • Water training	Work-, hobby-, or sport-specific movements at slow speed; emphasize coordinating upper- and lower-body movements.
Tuesday (easy)	*Morning* • ROM stretches, slow and luxurious! *Evening* • ROM stretches	*Choose one* • Water program *or* • Cycling *or* • Upper-body exercises	**Imagery** Watch a game. Appreciate movement away from the ball. ROM stretches while doing this.
Wednesday (hard)	*Morning* • ROM stretches • Level A exercises *Evening:* • ROM stretches • Level B exercises	*Choose one* • Elliptical *or* • Cycling *or* • Water training	Air tennis, air basketball, air golf, etc., can be "played" with a racket or club but without a ball. Happy feet.
Thursday (easy)	*Morning* • ROM stretches • Level A exercises *Evening* • ROM stretches	*Choose one* • Water training *or* • Upper-body exercises	**Imagery** Get yourself in a passive stretch position. Close your eyes and for 20 minutes feel, smell, hear, and see any sport.

(continued)

DAY	EXERCISE	TRAINING	MOVEMENT PATTERNS
Friday (hard)	*Morning* • ROM stretches • Level A exercises *Evening* • ROM stretches • Level B exercises	*Choose one* • Elliptical *or* • Cycling *or* • Water training	Job simulation. Ball toss, shoot hoop, 7-irons, etc., but *easy* (see Chapter 12).
Saturday (easy)	*Morning* • ROM stretches • Level B exercises *Evening* • ROM stretches	• Stretch • Upper body	Find someone who is not competitive to play with. Any sport, 25–50% speed.
Sunday (off!)	ROM stretches	• Move around in water	Watch game while doing ROM stretches.

SAMPLE HARD DAY TWO WEEKS
(OR MORE) POST-OP

8:00 A.M.   Wake up!

Warm-up: Core, upper body, or well leg: total 5–10 min.

ROM stretches, slow. Concentrate!

Shower.

9:00 A.M.   Light breakfast of fruit, oatmeal, watered-down juice.

Put knee in passive extension position with ice and saddlebag/purse while eating.

10:00 A.M. 1st exercise session:

Warm-up: Level A or B, stationary bike or elliptical machine.

ROM stretches: 10 min.

Level A exercises: 15–20 min.

Cool down with ROM stretches: 10 min, plus 5 min stationary bike or elliptical.

Perform more complex movement patterns: Feel where your center of gravity is.

Muscle massage: 5 min.

Ice: 20 min; passive extension and heel slides while icing.

12:00 noon   Nap: 45 min.

Wake up and repeat 8:00 A.M. warm-up routine, ROM.

1:00 P.M.   Light lunch of sandwich with whole-grain bread, yogurt, and fluids.

(continued)

2:00 P.M.	Attend to work/family. Put your knee in either a straight or flexed position so you can be getting some rehab done at the same time. While you're on the phone, try the cat walk pose to get full extension. When you tire of that, do some single-leg balances.
3:30 P.M.	House cleanup. Waltz through the rooms like Ginger Rogers or Fred Astaire and find more stuff to throw away!
4:00 P.M.	2nd exercise session: After the house-work warm-up, give yourself a good stretch. Do your next exercise session similar to the morning's, though using Level B this time. At least two days a week, get in the pool for a water work-out.
6:30 P.M.	Evening news on TV.
7:00 P.M.	Healthy dinner.
8–10:00 P.M.	Massage, more ice, ROM stretches. At least one day a week, fill out your Muscle Quality Tracker (see Chapter 7) to decide what needs more emphasis.
10:00 P.M.	Read some poetry by D'Anne Bodman. Write in your journal or blog.
11:00 P.M.	Lights out.

I know what you're thinking: What about those of us who are busy with school or jobs? Keep in mind that the above schedule is truly the ideal. Do what you can daily, trying to hit at least something in all three prongs and, on your days off, treat yourself to the full monty.

PART THREE

TOTAL RECOVERY AND BEYOND

11

PRONG 1, LEVEL C

Six More Exercises for Life After
Knee Surgery

THE EXERCISES IN this chapter are again variations of what you already know from Levels A and B. Everyone should do these basic exercises regularly for the rest of their lives. These sorts of *resistive exercises* (using weights, bands, or just gravity resistance) are necessary for guarding against osteoporosis (weakening of the bones with age) and also for maintaining general fitness so you can lift groceries and shovel snow. Throwing in some core and upper-body lifts between these exercise sets will make things less monotonous and improve your overall fitness.

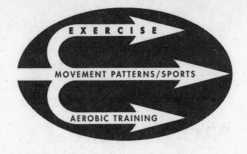

EXERCISE

MOVEMENT PATTERNS/SPORTS

AEROBIC TRAINING

DOUBLE-LEG SQUATS WITH DUMBBELLS

Purpose: To achieve maximum pumpitude by doing variations on the most important and functional exercise in the world, the squat. I know what you're thinking: been here, done this. Truth is, when it comes to the mother of all exercises, you can never do enough. The squatting motion is so much a part of your life—with gardening, sports, stairs, etc.—that you need to get these muscles as fit as possible.

Starting position: Stand with your feet shoulder-width apart, knees slightly bent, and quads and hamstrings already co-contracted. Keep back and arms straight with a dumbbell in each hand. You can use the stability ball or, better yet, do some reps with the ball and some reps without.

Action: Squat as if you are sitting in a chair. You can squat as far as you feel in control but not lower than 90 degrees at the knees. Keep your weight evenly distributed over both feet. Tempo = 2 seconds down/2 seconds up, *or slower*. Your lower back should feel strong and stable. Use a weight-lifting belt if you have one. Do 3 sets of 10 reps, three times a week.

Note: Men generally have more upper-body strength than women. Nevertheless, guys, if the heaviest thing you've lifted in the last twenty years is a beer, ten-pound weights may be too much for you at first. Dumbbells come in all different weights, so you can start low and work your way up.

Variations on the theme: I want you to really move *slowly* and increase the resistance (e.g., weight or heavier exercise bands) in Level C. To add more stress, hold your squat at the

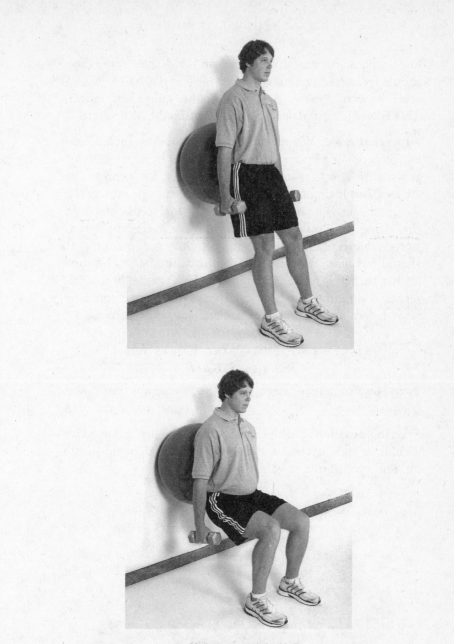

Double-leg squat with dumbbells

lowest point for as long as you can—and then some. You should feel a tremendous burn in your muscles by 15–30 seconds. As you get stronger, try to hold it longer and longer. This is where you make large gains in functional strength.

Superchallenge: When you are really good at squats, add biceps curls—a two-for-the-price-of-one exercise. Hold your arms, with weights, at your side. As you squat, bend at the elbows thus lifting the weight. Don't use a death grip on the weights. This is an arm exercise, and your biceps should do the lifting. As you stand, lower your arms. Triceps extensions while doing squats require more coordination but should feel natural for skiers. Obviously, squats can be done with a barbell instead of dumbbells. This necessitates a different technique and thus it is imperative that someone knowledgeable verifies your form and acts as a spotter.

Single-Leg Hamstring Curls with Stability Ball

Purpose: To increase strength of the hamstrings, hips, and back (the "core").

Starting position: Lie on the floor with one heel propped on a chair or stability ball and the other leg straight up in the air. Keep your arms at your sides for balance.

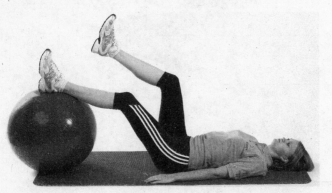

Single-leg hamstring curl

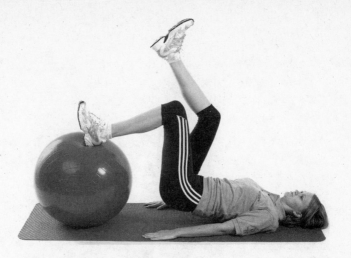

Single-leg hamstring curl

Action: When using a stationary object like a chair, push down on your heel while bending your knee and lifting your hips. When using a stability ball, get balanced and curl your heel toward your buttocks as far as you can. Return to the starting position in a controlled manner. Do not let your hips touch the ground between reps. Do 3 sets of 15 reps, *each leg,* three times a week.

Note: Using the stability ball takes some practice but it really challenges your balance, even while lying on your back. This is one of my favorite exercises as you can really feel it also working your core—the abdominal, back, and hip muscles.

LATERAL STEP-UPS WITH DUMBBELLS

Purpose: To move powerfully side to side while challenging balance and coordination.

Starting position: Standing next to a 3-inch-high box or step, start with light (5-pound) dumbbells.

Action: Step laterally onto the box and shift your weight completely to that leg. You should step with a slow, strong motion. Feel a good co-contraction as you straighten your knee without locking it into extension. Lower your opposite

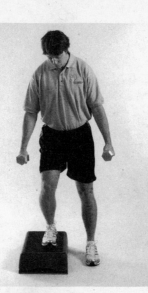

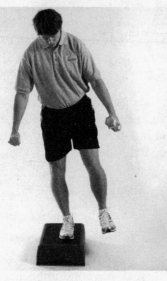

Lateral step-up with dumbbells

foot back to the floor slowly—do not just drop down. Do 3 sets of 10 reps, three times a week.

The key is not to push off the floor when stepping up, and to lower slowly on the way down.

Challenge: As you get stronger, increase the height you step up. Aim for a step of up to 10 inches or higher. Also increase the weight of the dumbbells.

FORWARD LUNGES

Purpose: A dynamic variation on the squatting theme, lunges are another functional motion that are part of everyone's life. Life does not stay in two dimensions, and neither should your exercises.

Starting position: Stand with your legs shoulder-width apart.

Action: Step (lunge) forward onto one foot while keeping the back foot on the floor. The majority of your weight moves with your front foot. Push off your front foot and

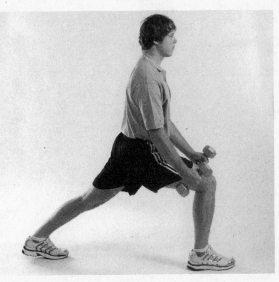

Forward lunge

return to the starting position. Do all 6 reps before switching legs. Make small lunges at first, slowly progressing to a lunge where the knee is bent 90 degrees *and your heel is directly below your knee*. For balance, put your hands on your hips, or hold your arms straight out at your sides. This can be a tough exercise, so start with 2 sets of 6 reps, three times a week. As you improve, add dumbbells, starting with 5 pounds.

I recommend doing lunges next to a mirror, so you can check your form—at least until you get the hang of it. Your knee should *never* bend past your heel.

LATERAL LUNGES

Purpose: To safely introduce coordinated lateral (side-to-side) motions, keeping strong and balanced.

Starting position: Stand with your legs shoulder-width apart, knees slightly bent, hands forward, and head up (the ready position).

Action: Step (lunge) to the side, putting the majority of your

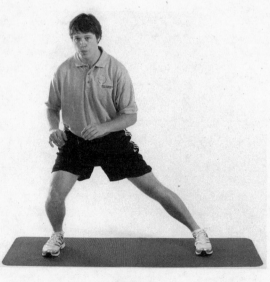

Lateral lunge

weight on the lunging leg. Maintain an erect upper body. Push off your lunging leg to return to the starting position. Switch sides. Begin with small steps. Just as the forward lunge, start slow with 2 sets of 6 reps, three times a week. Slow and strong!

Lunge as far as you can while maintaining good posture. Feel strong as you move back to the starting position. Begin with no weight and then add 5-pound dumbbells and increase the weight as you get stronger. Watch yourself in a mirror and correct your form. You should look like an athlete.

SINGLE-LEG BENCH SQUATS WITH DUMBBELLS

Purpose: Yet another variation on the squatting theme.

Starting position: Stand in front of a bench or chair. Put one leg up and leave the other leg slightly bent.

Action: While holding dumbbells, perform a single-leg squat while maintaining an upright position with a strong back. Tempo=2 seconds down/2 seconds up *or slower*. Feel a good stretch in the hip of the "up" leg.

Variations: Take a large step away from the bench to get into the starting position. Besides the TV, another trick to avoid rushing your exercises is to use a metronome (seriously—the one on the piano). I recommend 4 seconds for each rep (2 seconds up and 2 seconds back), but doing some reps slower is better still. The next variation is to do 5 reps very slowly, 5 reps slowly, and 5 reps fast (but controlled!).

Another variation is to change your body position by leaning forward as though you are looking for something on the ground. Do this with lighter weight than when your back is upright.

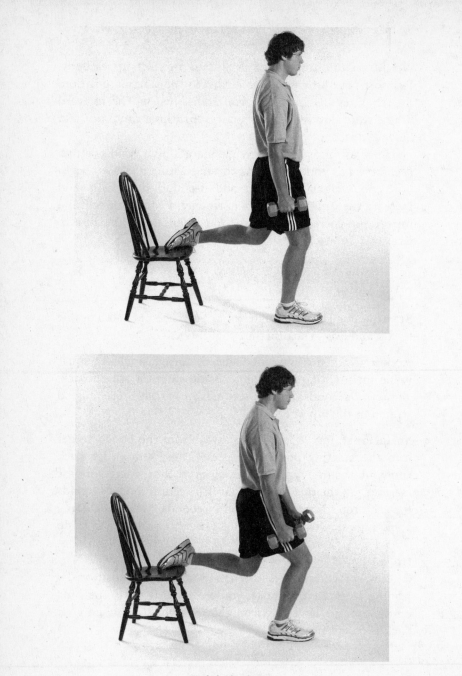

Single-leg bench squat

Getting Better than Before:
An Agenda of Health and Perseverance

Diligence is the mother of good fortune.
—*Don Quixote*

[There are worse things to be accused of than stubbornness. In the previous chapters I asked you to channel various athletes, but now I'm asking you to channel a stubborn mule extraordinaire (as well as one of my Irish brethren), Ernest Shackleton. Shackleton was the antarctic explorer whose entire crew survived over one year on a small island after their ship, the *Endurance*, was crushed by surrounding ice. The explorers survived essentially by strength of will (as well as by eating some less fortunate seals and penguins). I'm not here to tell you that "sometimes nothin' is a real cool hand," but I am saying that perseverance and stubbornness can serve you well in your recovery from misfortune, including the misfortune of an injured knee.

Let's look at some positives. You have survived not only the pain of surgery, but more significantly the annoyance, the inconvenience, and the feeling of mortality that often accompany this adventure. So,

give yourself a pat on the back.

You deserve it for all your hard and often boring work. However, that work is not quite over. Furthermore, now you must not consider it work but a lifestyle. As a football coach once said as I whined my way out of the weight room early one morning, "You think you're doing this because you need to, but you're actually doing this because you like it." And he was right. The weight did feel good to my bones and muscles. Revving *my* engine early in the morning kept me going the rest of the day. My mind might not like getting up at 5 A.M., but my body loved it. I hope you have begun to feel that love. Sure, it can be difficult to make time for exercise each day, but what is the alternative? To be an anchor with a bad knee the rest of your life? I think not.

THE LIFE OF A HEALTHY KNEE

Healthy knee people, one of whom you have now become, are plodding, predictable folk. They are cranky when they do not get their daily dose of exercise. They look for healthy things to eat on the lunch line. They swoon looking at the latest Patagonia catalog. They plan a vacation thinking of what they can do that is fun and active during the day. Sure they have their cannoli moments, but ultimately, they want to be healthy.

Here are some tips for moving forward with your *health-seeking knee*.

Keep a Training Manual

Way back in Chapter 2, I discussed goals and the importance of writing them down. A training manual can double as a date book, a calendar, or a personal organizer. The important thing is to create a written document of where you have been and what you have been doing. Some athletes are very elaborate in their daily entries, including information such as the weather, their body weight, their energy level, hours slept, food consumed, the perceived level of exertion of the workout, etc. But most of us will just make a quick notation such as

- Yoga (1 hour)
- Walk with a friend after lunch (30 min)
- Knee exercises (20 min)

By writing things down, you get an idea each week of how much time you spent doing something active. The goal for a health-seeking missile with a fully recovered knee should be at least five hours a week. Don't give yourself credit for wandering outside with your dog unless you are actually walking for fitness—getting your heart rate up and breaking a sweat. Do not make the training manual another burden on your day; use it as confirmation of your diligence.

Make a Sunday Night Training Plan

As you have learned by now, you need to build exercise into your life. Sit down on Sunday during *60 Minutes,* or at some point during the week, and put "me" time into your schedule just as you put in your kid's ball games, your business meetings, your food shopping, etc. People who cannot find even thirty minutes a day for themselves have their pants on fire. *Everybody* has thirty minutes on most days. Those thirty minutes are important not just to your knee's health but also to your overall well-being. The best spouses, the best workers, the best parents, the best anything all find time for themselves. Yes, it takes some thought and some juggling and sometimes you won't be able to fulfill your plan, but if you don't try it will never get done. And then nobody will be happy.

Hard Days, Easy Days

Your weekly plan should not be the same old, same old. As you schedule your week, think about how much time you have and where you will be. Are you passing the state park with that delivery on Thursday? Great, stop and power-hike up the trail. Is the weather report terrible? Catch an aerobics or Jazzercise class. This doesn't work into your schedule? Do a video workout at home while supper is on the stove. Whatever your plan, schedule *hard* and *easy* days. For example, you might consider that hike a hard workout, so the next day make it a soft workout, such as water aerobics or an easy bike ride and stretch. Weight workouts are almost always considered hard and should be done only three days a week unless you are careful to alternate muscle groups (e.g., legs on Monday, Wednesday, and Friday; core and shoulders on Tuesday and Thursday). The hard/easy days not only make things more interesting, but they also allow you to recover and keep you from burning out. Remember:

$$FITNESS = MOVEMENT + REST$$

By giving yourself the rest (easy days or soft workouts), you allow your body to repair and thus give you the fitness you are aiming for.

Change Your Workout Every Eight Weeks

Doing the same workouts week after week, year after year is not just boring for you mentally, it's also boring for you physically. Always repeating the same effort does not allow you to improve. Your body adapts to the same weight, the same movement patterns, the same walking course at the same pace, the same anything. You can see an example of this with strollers—folks who make the effort to go for a walk but never actually break a sweat. Humans are pretty efficient at walking and actually burn little energy doing it. As a result, if you use walking (or anything, for that matter) for activity, you need to make an effort, especially as your body adapts and gets more efficient.

Don't be a stroller! The folks at the gym without sweat on their brow, reading as they pedal the bike, are basically wasting their time. If you make the effort to go to the gym, go for a walk, or get in the pool—make it worth your while! Getting your heart rate up and breaking a light sweat are indications that you are working sufficiently in your training to produce health benefits for your muscles and your cardiovascular system.

What this might look like in the weight room is spending an eight-week block of doing, say, 10 reps and 3 sets of your exercises. After these eight weeks, raise the weight to where you can do only 6 reps, and perhaps increase the number of sets. Then in the next eight-week block, try 20 reps and only 2 sets with a lighter weight (as this increases strength *and* endurance). Bottom line: Once your knee has recovered, meet with a personal trainer (see Resources) to develop workouts that suit you and your *health-seeking* lifestyle.

The Winter of Your Discontent

I tend to discourage runners who aspire to anything more than a 10-K race. This is because any activity that is repetitive tends to cause overuse injuries. People in warmer climates are particularly vulnerable, as they are not limited by the elements. They can play baseball, golf, and tennis, and run year-round. The weather forces those of us in the North to adjust our activities, essentially cross training by default.

Unfortunately, the ice and snow also push some of us inside to vegetate for four months. Don't let this happen! Invest in snowshoes, shoe cables (e.g., Yaktrax, see Resources), fat bike tires, headlamps, skis, and terrific new clothes that make activity in cold weather fun and comfortable. There is no bad weather, just bad attitudes. You can't change the weather, so you might as well embrace it (and be glad you were not with Shackleton in Antarctica!).

12

RETURN TO SPORTS AND COMPETITION

For the Athlete in All of Us

SOME OF YOU might have skipped ahead from earlier chapters. Welcome! Because none of you are on the same time line, many things in this chapter can be done early in your three-pronged attack. Take a look at the following programs and perhaps ask your therapist or trainer how they might fit into your own knee's schedule.

Generally, at this stage in your rehab you should be comfortable with the *exercises* described in Levels A and B and have started to add in the variations from Level C. You have also been practicing simple *movement patterns* for your job and favorite sports to maintain muscle memory and doing the *aerobic training* at least at Level B (see Chapter 8). It is now time to ready yourself for something I like to call "normal life." The tricky part is when to start these more aggressive programs. In addition to seeking the opinion of your medical team, ask your knee. As a rule, these programs can start when you are walking at a normal speed with no pain and no limp. Not to tie you to any specific schedule, but ballpark figures (you could be ready sooner or later) for beginning the return to sport and competition programs are

- Arthroscopy: 3 weeks
- ACL reconstruction: 6 weeks
- Total knee replacement: read on

This stage of your rehab is truly the sharp end of the three-pronged attack. Use the return to sports programs in combination with your exercises and aerobic training to move to the next rung on the ladder: return to competition! The following are only suggestions, but they should give you an idea of the progression I want you to consider for all the activities you return to. Write out your own programs for Return to Firefighting, Return to Cross-Country Skiing, Return to Dog Grooming, etc. This is a worthwhile exercise for your psyche and your knee, and reinforcement for the healthy habits you want to continue.

A caution: Most of you will progress to do all of the activities you desire. Some of you, although you are able, should *never* do some things. For example, total knee replacement patients and other cartilage replacement patients would be better off *never* returning to running or aggressive pounding

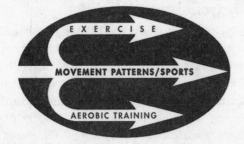

sports such as basketball or singles tennis. Ultimately, this is your decision, but make sure you broach the subject with your surgeon.

General Principles for a Return to Sports

Regardless of what sport or activity you are returning to, the progression is the same:

- Simple to complex
- Easy to hard
- Perfect movement patterns → change speeds → increase volume

RETURN TO RUNNING

Goal: To get back to running outside with no pain or swelling in the knee.

Like it or not, running is an aspect of almost all activities, so you must practice it, just not to excess. Ideally, you already started your Return to Running in the pool and on the treadmill with the aerobic program in Chapter 8. Remember that treadmill speeds are individualized and depend on stride length and running experience. Make sure you are familiar with the machine before pushing any buttons. When in doubt, proceed at a slower speed.

You can perform the following running workouts 3 days per week, staying at each level for a *minimum* of 1 week. You can also do some of the other return to sports programs while you are progressing in this one. If you have pain or swelling, RICE and go down one level until the swelling resolves.

This is another opportunity to tell you that running is not the only path to fitness. In fact, long-distance running—more than 3–5 miles, 3 days a week—is probably not the best thing for your joints. Addicted runners should make an effort to include some soft workouts such as cycling and water in their repertoire. Marathons might best be experienced as a course marshal.

Again, let's review the ballpark numbers for Return to Running, knowing there are some of you who will be earlier and some later:

- Arthroscopy: 3 weeks
- ACL reconstruction: 6 weeks
- Total knee replacement: I'm going to say not yet, knowing that your surgeon might say never (and I would probably agree). This is something the two of you will have to discuss.

LEVEL A

PURPOSE	Build off the treadmill walking program. Introduction to jogging.
PROTOCOL	Warm up with sit-ups or upper-body weights.
	Find a road or smooth trail with a slight uphill.
	Walk at brisk pace: 2 min
	Jog at slow speed: 1 min
	Repeat 4 times: 12 min
	Total: 15 min
COMMENTS	• Ideally you are comfortable with Level C of the treadmill walking program (see Chapter 8).
	• Jog UP an incline, walk DOWN.
	• If possible, spin (low resistance) on a bike for 5 min after jogging.
	• Ice your knee and stretch your entire lower leg when done.
	• If using a track, try jogging the straight and walking the curve.

LEVEL B

PURPOSE	Build on efficient movement patterns plus endurance.

PROTOCOL	Warm up with sit-ups and a brisk walk.	
	Walk at brisk pace:	1 min
	Jog at slow or medium speed:	3 min
	Repeat 4 more times:	**Total:** 20 min

COMMENTS
- Save time for a good cooldown in the water or on the bike, followed by stretching and ice.
- Remember, you may not be stressing your cardio system, but you are stressing your knee.
- After doing this for the first time, plan on a soft workout tomorrow, preferably in the water.
- Treat yourself to a professional massage.

LEVEL C

PURPOSE	Build endurance and coordination.

PROTOCOL	Warm up on the bike or with a brisk walk (5% incline if still using a treadmill).	
	Walk at fast pace. Stop and stretch quads and hams:	2 min
	Jog at a medium speed:	5 min
	Repeat 3 more times:	21 min
		Total: 28 min

COMMENTS
- Continue to avoid going downhill if running outside.
- If you don't spin on a bike or get in the water after jogging, at least cool down walking.
- Stretch, emphasizing the quads and hamstrings.
- Ice the knee and give it a good massage.

Progression Beyond Level C for the Running Addict

Once you are doing something similar to the Level C program, most of you serious runners will be keen to get back to your normal routine. *Resist that urge!* Continue on a gradual program similar to the one below and use the things that should now be habits: warming up, stretching, cooling down, hydrating, etc. Be methodical, but do not be afraid to miss a day. Spend anywhere from one to two weeks at these levels:

Level D: Jog 10 min *up* an easy grade, walk down and repeat once or twice. Start with three days a week.

If using a treadmill, increase the incline to 10 percent while jogging, and drop it to 5 percent during recovery walking. Once outside, it is worth the effort to find a cooperative hill.

Level E: Jog 15 min one day, 25 min the next. At least one day a week off.

Level F: Jog 20 min one day, 30 min the next. At least one day a week off.

Level G: Jog 20 min one day, 35 min the next. At least one day a week off.

Level H: Jog 20 min one day, 40 min the next. At least one day a week off.

After following a program such as this, you can work back into your usual training. This weekly progression would be common for an arthroscopic meniscus operation but might have to be stretched out for anything more complicated, such as an ACL reconstruction. Again, listen to your doctor and your knee. TKR patients should never run aggressively on the road.

Do not hesitate to repeat a week and progress only to a level where you feel comfortable. Pay close attention to the things I've discussed, plus proper running shoes, adequate orthotics (shoe inserts), warm clothes (what is it with runners in shorts in the middle of winter?), etc.

Make a weekly plan to schedule your runs and exercise. That's what Sunday night is for!

RETURN TO SOCCER

Goal: To rehabilitate your knee
while finally learning to *bend it.*

INJURY=OPPORTUNITY. Coming back from an injury or surgery provides an opportunity for you to work on fundamental skills. Have a new ball waiting for you the day you come home from the hospital. Start rolling it under your feet and up the wall those first days post-op while doing co-contractions and leg raises with co-contractions (see Chapter 3). As you progress through the exercises and aerobic training, spend time on simple, low-stress skills with the ball. Push it around the house. Be the ball.

You can perform each level of the Return to Soccer program three to four days per week alternating with soft workouts on the other days. You probably need to spend two weeks to perfect your technique at each level (though it may seem painfully slow, this is not the time to rush). If you have pain or swelling: RICE and go back one level until the swelling resolves. Quick step run with the ball at first (see Chapter 3) before progressing to a jog (see Return to Running earlier in this chapter).

While you watch games on TV and at the park, visualize yourself physically and mentally reacting to the flow of the game. Watch players moving without the ball. Think like Beckham. What would he see?

LEVEL A

PURPOSE	Body balance and coordination. Ball skills.
PROTOCOL	Warm up on the bike or with a fast walk. ROM stretches.

(continued)

Dribble while walking or easy jogging:	10 min
Wall taps (light):	3 min
Repeat 1 time:	13 min
	Total: 26 min

COMMENTS
- Use a lighter ball, if possible.
- Use any open space for dribbling (must be flat, no obstacles). Avoid gardens and dogs.
- Wall taps: Stay within 2 feet of the wall. Gently tap ball against the wall. Try to establish a rhythm with both feet.
- Stretch the entire lower body and ice the knee after the workout.

LEVEL B

PURPOSE Forgetting which foot is dominant.

PROTOCOL Warm up on the bike.

Dribble while easy jogging:	3 min
Partner passing:	10 min
Wall taps (light):	2 min
Repeat 1 time:	15 min
	Total: 30 min

You can do this drill 2 times a day, but since this is more aggressive than it seems, start with once a day and see how your knee responds.

COMMENTS
- Keep using the lighter ball.
- Stay slightly on toes while dribbling. Keep the ball close to your body.
- Wall taps: Maintain a rhythm. Use both feet!
- *Easy* passes with a friend.
- Ice your knee and have a good stretch.
- Try using a soft knee sleeve.

LEVEL C

PURPOSE	World Cup prep.
	Channeling Pelé.

PROTOCOL	Warm up.	
	Partner passing:	5 min
	Partner juggling:	2 min
	Cone dribbling (6–8 cones): up and back with ball, then up and back without ball:	10 min
	Drop-kick to wall, 50–70% effort:	3 min
	Repeat 1 time:	20 min
	Total:	40 min

Start with once a day for this drill. Move to twice a day if knee is doing well.

COMMENTS	• Switch to a regulation ball.

- Switch to a regulation ball.
- More aggressive partner passing: Stay on your toes, keep the ball close to your body.
- Juggling: Use your feet, knees, chest, and head. Keep the ball close to your body.
- Cone dribbling: Spread them out over 20 meters.
- Always perform exercises with both feet.
- Drop-kick: Hold ball in hands, release, and strike forward with proper kicking mechanics.
- Use the rebounds from the wall as an opportunity for fast trapping and ball control work.
- Cooldown and ice!

Return to Competition

- You should complete Level C successfully.
- Two-on-two or three-on-three games on a good surface are a great place to start game simulation training. No aggressive contact! Your teammates should apply passive defense until you are stronger and up to speed. Refuse to play with

knuckleheads who can't pull up on a tackle. Wear a red shirt or pinny to remind them you are rehabilitating.

- The Return to Running program is part of your Return to Soccer program, so review that section earlier in this chapter.
- Games: Start with 10–15 minutes on the field per half and take advantage of halftime to stretch and ice. This can be advanced to 20 minutes per half, and increase from there. Do not play your first returning game in the mud!

RETURN TO TENNIS

Goal: To get back on the court and use tennis
to rehabilitate your knee. At the same time, to use your
repaired knee to rehabilitate your tennis game.

INJURY = OPPORTUNITY. Coming back from an injury or surgery allows the opportunity for you to correct bad habits. Have your racket within reach when you return from the hospital. By day two post-op you should be standing and making easy strokes to maintain your muscle memory and to eliminate that vase you never liked. As you progress through your recovery, you should be spending time on simple, low-stress skills with the racket both on and off the court. Think footwork (quick step running in Chapter 3) and eye-to-hand coordination in these early weeks post surgery. Getting a coach or tennis savvy friend involved early in your rehab would ease your return.

Stay at each level for about two weeks. You can perform each level of the Return to Tennis program three to four days per week alternating with soft workouts on the other days. If you have pain or swelling, RICE and go back one level until the swelling resolves. Think about what makes Federer so good.

LEVEL A

PURPOSE   Balance and coordination.

Stroke/serve movement patterns.

Letting the knee know what you
plan to do in the coming days.

PROTOCOL   Warm up on the bike or with a walk.

1-step forehand and backhand:	2 min
Soft serve:	1 min
Repeat 4 more times:	12 min
	Total: 15 min

COMMENTS
- Ideally someone is tossing (not hitting!) the balls in position for you to swing smoothly.
- Start in the ready position when simulating forehand and backhand strokes. Return to the ready position and step into the next stroke.
- Concentrate on the toss and footwork on your serves. Striking the ball is of less importance.
- You can be doing these same exercises as *simulations* as soon as 2 days after surgery.
- Ice and stretch afterward.

LEVEL B

PURPOSE   Skills, game simulation.

Looking good in whites.

PROTOCOL   Warm up on bike or treadmill.

Volley, without and with ball:	3 min
Repeat 5 more times, with 1 min rest between sets:	**Total:** 23 min

COMMENTS
- Volley simulation using a racket but not a ball. This means moving right, left, forward, and backward. The emphasis is on quality of movements, not speed. Begin by just walking through this simulation.

(*continued*)

- Have a partner toss you some balls. Gently play them back with controlled lateral efforts.
- Advance to gentle wall volleys with a bounce (10 yards away) and work up to wall volleys with no bounce (5 yards away). Have a basket of balls so you're not chasing.
- Remember to do a proper cooldown, hydrate, and ice afterward.
- If you feel great, add another 23-min session after a rest—*but that's it!* Do not stay on the court until your knee is screaming.

LEVEL C

PURPOSE	Thinking about Wimbledon. Partner skills.

PROTOCOL	Warm up on the bike or treadmill.	
	Off-court warm-up: game simulation moving with the racket but not the ball:	5 min
	Net volley:	5 min
	Midcourt volley:	5 min
	Baseline volley:	10 min
	On-court movement: net, mid-, baseline, and serves:	5 min
		Total: 30 min
	Repeat once if the knee feels *great*.	

COMMENTS	• When volleying, stay in the center of the court. This not the time for extreme lateral movements.
	• Select a partner who is willing to play rehab tennis with you (someone who is pretty good and can keep the ball within your reach).
	• A well-planned and consistently implemented warm-up is critical for postinjury athletes. To do this you must arrive early!
	• Follow a proper cooldown program complete with stretching and icing.
	• HAVE FUN! Focus on movement, not victory.
	• Sign up for that lesson if you haven't already.

Return to Competition

Your return to competition progression, once you're comfortable with the above program, should look something like this:

Level D: 1 set, 50–75% intensity
Level E : 2 sets, 50–75% intensity
Level F : 3 sets, 50–75% intensity
Level G: 1 set, 75%; 1 set, 100%
Level H: 2–3 sets, 100%

Move up one level when you are feeling *great*, not just good. Spend at least two weeks at each level for experienced players, more than two weeks for most of us.

RETURN TO BASKETBALL

Goal: To be like Mike as quickly and safely as possible.

After years of working in sports medicine, it has become clear to me that basketball players have a genetic defect that does not allow them to warm up properly. They think the warm-up is tossing in a few layups. Luckily, special drugs used during your surgery have now corrected this defect. One great thing about basketball is the nice smooth surface it is played on. As a result, you can get on the court quickly. You cannot, however, get back to grabbing rebounds with five players hanging on you before your knee is ready. Follow the program and remember: You now have the ability to warm up, stretch, and cool down like all other athletes.

INJURY=OPPORTUNITY. Coming back from an injury or surgery allows you opportunity to emphasize fundamental skills that might need attention (e.g., foul shooting). There is no reason you can't be dribbling a basketball off the side of the couch with your nondominant hand the day you get back from the hospital (except it may drive your housemates crazy). Also set up that Nerf basket or just flip over a Tiffany lampshade.

You can perform each level of the Return to Basketball program three to four days per week alternating with soft workouts on the other days. You probably need to spend two weeks to perfect your technique at each level (though it may seem painfully slow, this is not the time to rush). If you have pain or swelling, RICE and go back one level until the swelling resolves. Quick step run with the ball at first (see Chapter 3) before progressing to a jog (see Return to Running earlier in this chapter).

Watch games on TV and at the gym. Imagine yourself physically and mentally reacting to the flow of the game. Watch players moving without the ball. Think like a point guard. Where is the ball going next?

LEVEL A

PURPOSE	Remembering the smell of the gym. Ball skills.
PROTOCOL	Warm up with your new abilities.
	Stationary dribbling, eyes closed, change hands: 5 min
	Walk and dribble, move forward and backward: 10 min
	Repeat 1 time: **Total:** 30 min
COMMENTS	• Standing and dribbling can start in the house a few days after surgery.
	• In the gym, stay away from blockheads who do not understand you are recovering from surgery.
	• Consider using the pool for shot simulation. Find a water hoop.
	• Cool down, stretch, and ice.

Level B

PURPOSE	Seeing the whole of the moon. Shooting and passing skills.

PROTOCOL   Warm up on the bike.

Skills

Standing layups (both sides!):	5 min
8' perimeter field goals:	5 min
One-step passing:	10 min
Repeat 1 time:	20 min
	Total: 40 min

COMMENTS
- Low-intensity jumping in Level B. Use your calves and hips as shock absorbers.
- Stationary dribble and shoot, or receive a pass and shoot.
- Stationary or one-step when passing but feel some bounce in your knees.
- You can show up to practice, but do not shoot with the team or participate in moving drills yet.
- Stretch and ice.

Level C

PURPOSE	Improving shooting and ball skills. Remembering that Bird is the word.

PROTOCOL   Warm up properly.

Moving layups:	5 min
Medium perimeter field goals:	10 min
Free throws:	10 min
Dribbling drills: Emphasize an athletic position, quick hand work:	15 min
All-team *drills* (not scrimmages) at medium speed, controlled:	30 min
	Total: 70 min

(continued)

COMMENTS
- Arrive early and take time to warm up. This is key for all athletes but especially those returning from injury.
- Medium intensity jumping in Level C.
- Ball skills should increase in intensity.
- You can move about the court with your teammates, but they should remember you are recovering from knee surgery so wear a red shirt or pinny.
- Cooldowns are just as important as warm-ups.
- The pool is a great place to work out stiffness.
- Stretch and ice.

Return to Competition

Your return to competition progression should look something like what follows. The important thing is to find someone who will work *with* you, not against you. Plan on at least one week at each of the following levels combined with skill work (such as in Level C), exercises, and aerobic training.

Level D: 1-on-1: low intensity, minimal contact (15–20 min)
Level E : 2-on-2: medium intensity (20–30 min)
Level F : 3-on-3: full court, medium to high intensity
Level G: Full team: 5 min in, 5 min out

How quickly you proceed with this model progression depends on how both your surgeon and your knee feel. You must be able to pull back the intensity and concentrate on your basketball skills. Enter scrimmages with a red shirt and don't make your first game against your team's archrival. Your first game experience should be "garbage time" to get your mojo working.

RETURN TO
BASEBALL/SOFTBALL

Goal: To rehabilitate your knee on the field
while correcting previous bad habits.

Within days of your surgery, I want you to practice movement patterns from the ball field that will additionally serve to rehabilitate your knee. Get into your batting stance and step into a pitch. See the ball—visualize the pitcher's release point. Now try the same thing with fielding a fly ball. Put on a glove and follow the imaginary ball coming in. Take an easy stride as you toss it back to the infield. Doing these simple visualizations will really make a difference until you're ready to get outside.

Feedback from a knowledgeable coach is especially important in sports that use both upper and lower extremities, as it can be that much easier to get into bad habits. Remember, nothing ruins shoulders faster than weak legs! Rotator cuff exercises and other upper-body exercises are key for every throwing athlete but especially those returning from injury.

You can perform each level of the Return to Baseball program three to four days per week alternating with soft workouts on the other days. You probably need to spend two weeks to perfect your technique at each level (though it may seem painfully slow, this is not the time to rush). If you have pain or swelling, RICE and go back one level until the swelling resolves. Quick step run at first (see Chapter 3) before progressing to a jog (see Return to Running earlier in this chapter).

Watch games at the park or on TV with an eye toward player patterns—how the pitcher works a batter or how good fielders position themselves. Visualize yourself on the field and mentally react to the flow of the game as a smarter player. Remember, you no longer see the old you. You now see the new and improved you: the Jackie Robinson–reincarnated you.

LEVEL A

PURPOSE	Light toss. Swing simulation.

PROTOCOL	Warm up on the bike.

Shoulder strengthening with stretch bands.

Play catch with a partner, about 20':	5 min
Step forward and throw 40' (light effort):	5 min
Simulate full swing with a light bat:	2 min
Repeat 1 time if feeling great:	12 min
Total:	24 min

COMMENTS

- All throws with a partner need to be light.
- Think about starting the throw with your legs and your core.
- Avoid sudden lateral movements to catch the ball.
- Stretch and ice the knee (and shoulder) after the workout.
- When was your last eye appointment? Now's a good time.

LEVEL B

PURPOSE	Channeling Willie and the Babe.

Light toss, grounders.

Bat swings with tee.

PROTOCOL	Warm up on the bike.

Shoulder strengthening with stretch bands.

Catch and throw easy:	2 min
Step forward and throw (medium speed):	10 min
Take some grounders at a slow speed:	10 min
Easy swings with a batting tee:	5 min
Repeat 1 time if feeling great:	27 min
Total:	54 min

COMMENTS
- Your throws to your partner can be faster than Level A, but stay focused on accuracy. Increase the distance of the throws to 60'.
- Avoid sudden lateral movements to catch the ball.
- Work on proper mechanics for catching slow ground balls. Ready position → squat → scoop → set → throw. Do your knees bend?
- Cool down in the water if possible. Bring an old bat and do some harder swings underwater.

LEVEL C

PURPOSE
Working on weaknesses.
Grounders, batting practice.

PROTOCOL
Warm up.
Shoulder strengthening with stretch bands.

Skills

Vary catch and throw from 20' to 90', slow to fast:	5 min
Take grounders at medium speed and begin lateral movements:	10 min
Swing at medium-speed pitches. Hit 10+ line drives up the middle:	10 min
Return to full practice at 50% speed initially. Advance to 100% over the next 3 weeks. Base running is allowed only if you have progressed to Return to Running Level C:	60 min
	Total: 85 min

COMMENTS
- Lateral movements and jogging after balls are now allowed.
- You can now enter the batting cage and take medium-speed pitches. This is the time to work on proper mechanics. Get some coaching!
- Cool down and ice.
- For Pete's sake, *no* feet-first sliding! Headfirst sliding is safer for your knees but requires practice.

Return to Competition

The nice thing about baseball is you can get yourself back into the games gradually: designated hitter with a pinch runner, one or two innings in the field, or one inning on the mound. What you must guard against is yourself. Are you the type of competitor who has to take out the catcher at home plate even if you're already ahead by nine runs? Do you have to slide every time? If so, you have to wait a bit longer before getting into games. Again, no one plays nine innings in spring training! You are in spring-training mode. A gradual, safe return is worth more than that tenth run.

RETURN TO ALPINE SKIING

Goal: To get you back on the slopes having fun and enjoying the fresh air. And by the way, you'll be rehabilitating your knee.

I will now attempt to slay the mythic beast of skiing and knee injuries. For more than a decade, I have allowed my experienced skiers to return to skiing as soon as they have the muscle control to do so. Actually, I do not let them ski, I let them *rehabilitate their knee on their skis*. This includes TKR and ACL reconstruction patients who can get on skis as early as six weeks post-op *if*

- they are experienced skiers.
- they have full motion and good muscles.
- there are good snow conditions.
- they follow the program below.
- they have someone skiing with them both to watch out for potential danger and criticize their technique. As I have said before, returning from injury is a great time to eliminate bad habits, but most of us need some coaching to do so.

In twenty years of practice, I have yet to experience a skier tearing his or her graft on the slopes in the first six months post ACL surgery. The same for TKR patients. Good skiers do not injure their knee in controlled skiing. They injure their knee in aggressive race situations or in recreational skiing when they are not paying attention. This does not mean you cannot reinjure your knee on the slopes, but in the controlled rehab period you are more apt to reinjure your knee on an icy parking lot than on the ski slopes (just be careful when walking to the lodge!). The key is to be strong and alphabetical: A to B to C.

You can perform each level of the Return to Skiing program three to four days per week, alternating with soft workouts on the other days. You probably need to spend two weeks to perfect your technique at each level (though it may seem painfully slow, this is not the time to rush). If you have pain or swelling, RICE and go back one level until the swelling resolves.

LEVEL A

PURPOSE	Balance and coordination. Return of "snow confidence."
PROTOCOL	Warm up on the bike or take a brisk walk. Take 6 runs on short skis and easy terrain (controlled speed, low intensity): **Total:** 90 min *Do not* ski 2 days in a row!
COMMENTS	• Warm up to ski, don't ski to warm up. • Rent a pair of short skis for the first weeks of skiing since at slow speeds short skis are easier to turn and less stressful on the knee. • Ski only on easy terrain (green) for the first two outings but avoid the carnage—and humiliation—of the bunny slope. • Cool down in a pool if possible. Stretch and ice.

(*continued*)

LEVEL B

PURPOSE	Feeling the inside edge. Technical skills.
PROTOCOL	Warm up on the bike or take a brisk walk. Take 8–10 runs on well-groomed trails. Your choice of skis: **Total:** up to 3 hours *Do not* ski 2 days in a row!
COMMENTS	• Keep the speed down and work the technical aspects of skiing (balance, stance, hands forward, etc.). • This is on-snow *rehab*. You must concentrate on every movement. Also, you must continue your programs of exercise and aerobic training. • If you're a racer, your coach needs to be involved at this stage. If you're not a racer, now is a great time to take a lesson. • Cool down, stretch, and ice.

LEVEL C

PURPOSE	Balance, strength, and endurance.
PROTOCOL	Warm up on the bike or take a brisk walk. Take 10–15 runs on firm, groomed trails. You can now ski the blue trails or the smooth black trails if you are an expert skier: **Total:** up to 4½ hours Racers: A gate training progression needs to be established with your coach.
COMMENTS	• Always take it easy on the first 2–3 runs. • Speeds should be natural and completely under control. • Turn frequently to work on technique, improve strength, and keep your speed under control.

- Stop skiing *before* you are fatigued. Take breaks, hydrate, and beware of deteriorating conditions and flat light.
- Avoid unpredictable conditions for the first year post-op (heavy wet snow, woods skiing, moguls, fog, etc.).
- Have you gotten that lesson yet?
- As always, cool down (in the pool if possible), stretch, and ice.

Return to Competition

While it's an easy decision letting someone on the slopes to rehab for the first time, getting back to competition is a bit tougher. Unlike softball, you cannot titrate your effort in a ski race. Gravity dictates your speed and the ruts dictate the difficulty. That said, this is one of those plans that must be made with the opinion of your coach, your knee, and your doctor. Once you've made the decision to race, you have to commit fully. When doing your race imagery, you should feel strong and excited—not nervous about crashing. If you have those thoughts, you might need a few more weeks of training.

RETURN TO GOLF

Goal: To lower your handicap while rehabilitating your knee.

Most golfers actually play better after a knee or shoulder injury. Want to guess why? Simply because they slow their swing! Although I talk about getting some coaching in my other sports programs, nowhere is it as important as when returning to golf. Get a lesson! Use the bad luck of knee surgery to improve your golf game.

You should have been swinging your 5- or 7-iron inside days after surgery while trying to model Tiger or Annika. In

other words, don't practice your same crummy swing—
make some adjustments! If you haven't been handling your
clubs, spend a few days doing this before hitting real balls.
You can perform each level of the Return to Golf program
three to four days per week, alternating with soft workouts
on the other days. You probably need to spend two weeks to
perfect your technique at each level (though it may seem
painfully slow, this is not the time to rush). If you have pain
or swelling, RICE and go back one level until the swelling resolves.

Upper-body and core exercises are crucial for golfers. Besides the lesson, taking a Pilates class is probably the best
thing you can do to improve your game.

LEVEL A

PURPOSE	A slower swing. Understanding greens.
PROTOCOL	Warm up.
	Stretch, including legs, back, shoulders.
	5-iron off tees. Easy, three-quarter swing. Hit 20–30 balls: 20 min
	Putting: 20 min
	Total: 40 min
COMMENTS	• Get a good stretch of not just your knee but also shoulders and back before and after hitting balls.
	• Pay attention to your weight shift. You are swinging slowly enough that you should *feel* exactly where you are.
	• Ice the knee afterward.

LEVEL B

PURPOSE	Feeling your hips and hands. Balanced stance.

PROTOCOL	Warm up legs, shoulders, and back.	
	Easy three-quarter swings with 4- through 9-irons. Use up to 100 balls:	75 min
	More putting:	15 min
	Total:	90 min
COMMENTS	• Continue using a three-quarter swing.	
	• Focus on striking the ball—no muscling.	
	• Stretch during; stretch and ice afterward.	

LEVEL C

PURPOSE	Channeling Babe Didrikson. Smelling azaleas.	
PROTOCOL	Warm up, full stretch.	
	Full swings with 4- through 9-irons. Use up to 100 balls. Add woods after 2 weeks of irons:	75 min
	Putting:	15 min
	Total:	90 min
COMMENTS	• How are those lessons going?	
	• Use breathing and flow, not strength.	
	• Full swing but still slow (think metronome).	
	• Hit the ball to feel good, not to beat your partner.	
	• Keep your neck and shoulders relaxed.	
	• Don't rush.	
	• Stretch and ice afterward.	

Return to Competition

The next objective and beyond is to get back on the course with a better game. Remember, you are rehabilitating your knee—not actually playing golf. Ergo, winter rules: (1) If it lands in a gully, take a drop; (2) use a cart for the first weeks; and (3) most important, do not keep score! Use this time to find out why you like golf—the fresh air, the companionship, the good cigars, the beautiful vistas, the nineteenth hole. Let your game improve with *deliberate practice*. Start with one good shot per hole and move on from there.

13
FREQUENTLY ASKED QUESTIONS

Sunbathing, Supplements, Getting
Back to Work, and More

IDEALLY, YOU SHOULD feel comfortable asking your health-care team member for advice and information about your recovery from knee surgery. However, since things can go pretty fast in a busy office, bring a list of questions and make sure they get answered. Unfortunately, if you are like most people, there's always something you've forgotten. This chapter is designed to help you with answers to some of the most common questions.

What type of anesthesia should I have for surgery?

If you are a healthy person, the type of anesthesia is actually up to you and the anesthetist. The basic choices are either a general anesthetic where you fall asleep or a spinal anesthetic where just your legs are numbed. If you have a spinal anesthetic, you can watch what is going on and can ask questions during the course of the operation (see Chapter 5). Some surgeons do a knee arthroscopy under local anesthesia like at the dentist. This is not my first choice, but it's something you can discuss with your doctor if the other options freak you out.

How often should I ice?

For the first week following a knee operation, icing is one of your main jobs. You should spend at least twenty minutes every two hours icing your knee. At minimum, you should do this five or six times a day. Do not forget also to elevate the knee while icing. As healing progresses, you will stop icing as often, but I recommend that you ice or use some icing system (e.g., Cryo/Cuff) after any hard workout for four to six months after surgery. (See Chapter 2 for more information on icing.)

How incapacitated will I be right after surgery?

For the first week, you'll spend much of your time with your knee elevated above the level of your heart. It should not be below heart level for more than fifteen minutes at a time except when you are doing your rehab. Arthroscopy patients can usually begin easing back to normal activities *in addition* to your rehab program by week two post-op. For ACL and TKR patients it is more complicated and covered extensively in this book.

If you have to get on the computer that first week, use a laptop propped on your belly while lying down. For the desktop crowd, limit computer time to fifteen minutes and follow that with an hour of proper elevation. Many people feel good after the first few days and are keen to get back to normal life. I caution you, however, to resist the temptation to jump right back into the fray. Take the time now to let your knee rest and heal properly, or you will set yourself up for a much longer, more painful recovery. (See Chapter 6 for more information on "the critical first week.")

When can I take a shower?

Many doctors are strict about this, so be sure to follow your doctor's advice. It is usually recommended to keep the knee(s) dry until the stitches are out. Whenever you are near water, wrap your knee with plastic wrap to cover the incisions. If the wounds get wet, dab them with a paper towel slopped with rubbing alcohol. After you are given the go-ahead to take a shower, place an old chair or stool in the tub to sit on until your strength and balance are back to normal. (Again, see Chapter 6.)

Why the focus on hydration? After all, I seem to be doing a lot of lying around.

You should drink plenty of fluids (preferably noncaffeinated) three to four days *before* surgery, much as you would hydrate before running a long race. Here's why: The minute you go into the hospital, they start pumping you with all sorts of medicines, sticking you with needles, and just generally causing you stress. If you show up hydrated, strong, and rested, your body is better prepared for this onslaught. After surgery, you are going to again be hydrating with the same watery sports drink or watery juice to help wash all these foreign chemicals out of your system. By drinking something other than plain water you will tend to drink more and also add some electrolytes that you lost during the stress of surgery.

If I drink a lot of milk, will I heal faster?

A nutritionally sound diet is important for general health, but there is no proof that drinking extra milk speeds healing in the short term, even for your bones.

That being said, I do encourage my patients to get adequate calcium in their diet, and one of the easiest forms of this is milk. If you suffer from lactose intolerance, you can get your calcium in other ways, including lactose-free milk products, tofu and other soy foods, almonds, supplements, and more.

What about taking supplements?

I recommend taking a multivitamin with iron both before and after surgery. While there is no direct proof that a supplement will help you heal faster, considering possible nausea from medications and the change in your diet around this time, taking a vitamin and mineral tablet is certainly reasonable. There is no evidence that glucosamine/chondroitin or other supplements marketed for arthritis help you heal or rehabilitate faster after surgery. They might have some benefit in long-term arthritis care, and you should discuss this with your doctor.

How can I decrease scarring?

Any scarring you have after your surgery predominantly has to do with genetics, where the incision is made, your health status at the time of surgery, and your aftercare of the wound. Keep the wound clean and dry until the stitches come out. Once the stitches are removed, gently apply a salve or lotion containing vitamin E twice a day. Vitamin E has been proved to be good for your skin and is now an ingredient in many products. Do not rub aggressively for the first month, as this may increase scarring. You can, however, rub in the *area* of the wound to desensitize and break up scar tissue. Your nurse or therapist will give you tips on this. Also, for the first year following surgery, use a sunblock of SPF 45 on all incisions to protect your vulnerable new skin from the sun.

Generally, I have not found any type of plastic surgery for knee scars to be particularly useful. How about this? Use your scar as a talisman for regular exercise and a physically fit lifestyle!

Do balms, herbs, and other remedies help in healing?

If someone wants to charge you a lot of money for a certain remedy but cannot show you legitimate studies of its effectiveness in a peer-reviewed journal (like the *New England Journal of Medicine* and other periodicals with editorial boards that scrutinize the articles submitted for publication), be careful. Always consult with a doctor or nurse before ingesting, applying, purchasing, or using products that sound too good to be true.

How will I know if I have an infection or other complication?

In the majority of cases, your body will tell you if something bad like an infection or other problem is developing. As long as you seem to be progressing (even if it is not as quickly as you would like), you are probably healing just fine. If you start to get worse, or especially if you feel sick (fever, chills, nausea), call your doctor right away. This is one of those subjects that we surgeons never like to think about, but complications do happen in a small number of cases. Potential complications are another reason why you must make sure the lines of communication are open with your doctor's office.

When will I be able to drive?

Driving may begin when you can comfortably enter and exit your car. That means usually within four or five days postsurgery for arthroscopic procedures, a week or two for ACL surgeries, and three or more weeks for TKRs. When you do start driving again, try it in a parking lot or on a quiet street at first, making sure there is no significant pain when you hit the brakes (or horn!).

When can I get back to work?

Return to work varies greatly from person to person, depending on the type of surgery you had and the type of job you do. Some *general* (and perhaps ideal) guidelines follow for arthroscopic surgery cases; most TKR patients need to *triple* the times listed below, and ACLs are somewhere in between.

- Return to a sedentary (sit-down) job may be as early as one week post-op for four hours a day.

- Two weeks after surgery, you may return to full-time light duty work. This consists of some walking at work—with crutches when needed—as long as it is inside and on a safe, flat surface. The majority of the day will still be sedentary.

- Three to four weeks post-op, continue full-time light duty with the sedentary hours decreasing. Whenever possible, ice and elevate the knee.

- A return to sports and heavy jobs (like construction, logging, and so forth) can take anywhere from two months for an arthroscopy to four months for an ACL to more than six months for a TKR.

- For more aggressive jobs, try to set up a gradual return-to-work program with your employer ahead of time. This could translate into limited hours as well as limited duty. In my opinion, you should not be stuck in the house with cabin fever just because people at work have said not to come back until you are "110 percent." Again, the question of returning to work is a highly individual one, but your boss, doctor, physical therapist, or trainer should be able to help you determine a reasonable program.

Swelling is never a good sign, right?

Right. Some swelling is from the water that was pumped in during the arthroscopy, some is from bleeding, and the rest is from fluid produced by cells inside your knee that were upset by the injury or surgery. Joints do not like to be swollen and stretched, so I want you to get rid of the swelling as quickly as possible. After you return to activities, swelling the next day will usually warn you that you did too much. Using a sleeve or wrap can help to hold down swelling and, contrary to tales from those old wives, will not make you dependent on one forever.

How will I know if I am exercising or working too much?

Your knee is not good at keeping secrets. You will be the first to know if you have overdone it because you will have pain and swelling the very next day. If you get a flare-up, whether it is at one week, one month, or one year postsurgery, take that day off, do some stretching and icing, and things should calm down. "Working through" swelling is usually a bad idea. Revisiting your RICE principles from Chapter 2, on the other hand, is an excellent idea. The very worst thing you can do is keep exercising to the point where you are losing range of motion. If that happens, contact your doctor, physical therapist, or trainer and get started immediately on the ROM stretches in Chapter 2.

Now that one knee has been operated on, should I worry about the other knee?

No—and yes. It all depends on what brought you to the doctor in the first place. If you suffered an injury on the football field, you're allowed to have pain in that knee. On the other hand, if you started having pain in one knee with no obvious trauma, it might be a genetic or age issue (e.g., arthritis) and could manifest in your other knee. The good news is that humans are not perfectly symmetrical: Just because you have something on one side doesn't mean you will have it

on the other. We all have a dominant hand and a dominant eye. A problem with one knee does not necessarily show up in the other.

How long will my arthroscopic/ACL/TKR surgery last?

If only your meniscus cartilage is damaged, your knee
should function pretty well for years to come. If you
also had some articular (surface) cartilage damage (that
is, early arthritis), you might be looking at more surgery in the next decade or so. No one has a crystal ball,
but I believe it is better to stay fit and have fun rather
than put yourself in a Barcalounger for the rest of your
life. Nowadays we have some other tricks, such as viscosupplementation (see Glossary), that might relieve
some arthritic symptoms. Ask your doctor about
these, but remember, nothing is as good as keeping
yourself in motion and staying healthy.

The success rate for ACL reconstruction in the
recreational athlete is in the 80 to 90 percent range. In
other words, you should be able to get back to most of
your activities without further injury to that ACL. Unfortunately, we know there is a higher incidence of
arthritis in these knees twenty or so years down the
road. This is why I tell almost of all of my ACL surgery
patients not to aspire to be marathon runners.

A total knee replacement is said to last fifteen
years or better, but this projection assumes that you
take good care of your new knee. Keeping your knee
for "activities of daily living" and not aggressive
sports will allow it to last longer (see Chapter 12 and
below).

**Which activities are *not* recommended after knee
surgery? What about skiing, softball, hockey, dancing,
golf, doubles tennis, and sex?**

This is always a tough question for the TKR patients,
so I will address the other patients first.

After any well-performed surgery short of a TKR, and a proper rehabilitation program, there is no reason you cannot get back to almost all of your sports, including the above. Most knee surgeries are about not only relieving pain but also returning to fun activities. If there is a reason your doctor does not want you doing certain sports, ask for an explanation. Anyone with significant surface (articular) cartilage damage should avoid participating in pounding activities—running, basketball, hard singles tennis, etc.—on any regular basis.

When it comes to the aggressive sports listed above, TKR folks must discuss this with their surgeon (preferably before the surgery). I recommend activities such as alpine skiing only for people who were already experts, and even then, I ask them to stick to the groomed trails. Hockey and softball should be played strictly for fun—not as a blood sport. Since singles tennis can be tough on your knees, easy doubles tennis is the most stress I recommend. As for dancing and golf: love them, but no Gene Kelly moves!

When it comes to sex, I would ask the gentle reader to use common sense and perhaps a bit of imagination.

Will I need to wear a brace the rest of my life?
First, let's distinguish between braces with metal and those without. For cartilage and TKR patients, your doctor will sometimes recommend a soft brace (no metal), also called a knee sleeve. A sleeve helps hold down swelling (which we have established is never a good thing), keeps your knee warm, and generally tells your knee that you care. You do not get dependent on a soft brace, so if you like one, use it with abandon.

I do not treat all of my ACL patients with a brace. But if you are an athlete or laborer on the fast track back to work or competition, I recommend wearing one during aggressive activities. Every doctor has a different opinion about bracing, and there are various studies that support both positions. In the majority of ACL cases, no brace is necessary after the first year or so, but again, if you feel more comfortable bracing for aggressive sports, go for it.

If you do choose to use a brace, whether hard or soft, it must fit properly. Do not borrow anyone else's brace without first checking with an athletic trainer or someone knowledgeable regarding brace fitting.

Will my knee ever be normal?

In a sense, your knee was not "normal" to begin with. That is, all knees have some wear and tear at just about any age. Our job as doctors and rehab folks is to help you do the things you want to do without pain. For the young people, it is also our job to make sure you do not ruin your knees for the future. It is hard to appreciate when you are twenty that you will someday be forty. Using the principles in this book and the advice from your doctor and trainer will go a long way toward making your knee "act normal." Unfortunately, everything—your car, your house, your teeth, and your knees—requires some maintenance.

Does everyone who has knee surgery need crutches?

Pretty much. You should be reasonably comfortable using crutches due to your injury, but if you haven't been on crutches (e.g., TKR patients), get a pair and practice before the surgery (see Chapter 4). Five minutes of practice walking with crutches will pay big dividends, particularly if you have surgery during the winter.

How much does my weight have to do with my knee problems?

One subject that comes up whenever we discuss knee injury and knee arthritis is obesity. Obviously obesity is not a good situation for any part of your body, but especially your joints. The more you weigh, the more stress you put on your knees. This means if you're over-weight, the sooner you do something about it the bet-ter. Getting fit is not just about dieting. In fact, it's probably not about dieting at all. It's about eating right and moving. Moving on arthritic knees of course is eas-ier said than done. If you can't even walk because of knee pain, you have to get imaginative. This is where water exercise (Chapter 9), my aerobic training pro-grams (Chapter 8), yoga, Pilates, and other nonpound-ing activities come into play. Get help. Get a personal trainer if possible. It's not just about the knee. It's about a healthy you.

What is the one best thing I could do to get my knee better as fast as possible?

You are doing the one thing—you're reading this book! Just as important, of course, is making sure you have good doctors, therapists, and trainers. Your genetics and your fitness state are hard to change in the short term. What you can do, and what I hope you'll get from this book, is pay attention to the details, or, in contrast to a much better-known author, learn to sweat the small stuff. The ice, hydration, exercises, a systematic approach to return to sports and work, training programs—this is what is going to get you better faster. I promise.

EPILOGUE

WHAT I HOPE you have noticed in the past weeks of knee rehabilitation is a general feeling of well-being. For the nonathletes, you are probably more in touch with your body than you have been for years. For the athletes, you have spent the time reconnecting with specific movement patterns and eliminating mistakes without the stress of competition. The ripples of health are flowing.

Do I really believe having knee surgery can change your life? Of course I do, and why wouldn't I? It takes so little to make positive changes in our lives. Think back to how fifteen minutes of housecleaning can change your attitude. This same principle applies to everything in this book. That last degree of motion, the small improvement in quad and hamstring strength, that two-second increase in single-leg balance are all quantitative measures of how much better you have become. Now, what if we put together that improved knee with a cleaner house and a healthier diet? We would have nothing less than a personal revolution!

While everyone talks about a mind-body connection in life, we really see few examples of this in practice. I hope I have been able to develop these connections for a faster and easier rehab. Additionally, using the three-pronged attack of exercise, movement patterns, and aerobic training in your post-rehab life will maintain the fitness habits you began while recovering. In the operating room I instruct everyone to sweat the small stuff because there is no small stuff. In your life there is no small stuff, either. Are you telling me that freshly laundered sheets you put on Sunday night don't feel great? Isn't the smile you get from your dog when you're heading out for a walk terrific? These are not big things alone, but they add up to what makes life worth living. Why do you think most "happiness" surveys find that, once you have food and shelter, money accounts for only 5 percent of "happiness"? That's because it's not the big stuff that matters—it's the small stuff. It's the phone call from your college roommate on your birthday. It's a line drive up the middle. It's the smell of the garden after the rain. It's the rock-hard feel of your quad muscles. Despite not having the greatest knees, you might actually be healthier than before all this started. Who would have guessed that a bad knee could turn into something positive?

RESOURCES

AT THE END of the day, only you can know what truly works best for your total recovery from surgery. Healing is a highly individual matter, and it is absolutely true that no two people are alike. To make your individual rehabilitation easier, the lists below cover a wide range of topics—to help you help yourself. The equipment list should allow you to locate some products that make rehab go easier. Moreover, items such as stability balls and weights will help you stay fit for life.

Feel free to contact me with any thoughts, suggestions, questions, or for a consultation:

www.THEALPINECLINIC.com

EQUIPMENT AND PRODUCTS

The following companies have many of the items discussed in this book. Any investment you make will be an investment in yourself and will pay dividends for years to come.

PERFORM BETTER

11 Amflex Drive
PO Box 8090
Cranston, RI 02920-0090
Phone: 1-888-556-7464
Fax: 1-800-682-6950
International phone: 401-942-9363
International fax: 401-942-7645
Web: www.performbetter.com
E-mail: performbetter@mfathletic.com

Lots of fun exercise/therapy equipment, such as
Biofoam roller. Used for massage and stretching the legs and back. Great for hamstring tendon ACL reconstructions.

Dyna Disc pillow. Used for balance training in Levels B and C of the exercise program.

Exercise bands. Can be used in place of dumbbells for exercises in Levels B and C and for shoulder exercises in Return to Baseball/Softball, Return to Golf.

Jump rope. Great for agility, coordination, and aerobic training.

Stability ball. Used in Levels B and C of the exercise program and for core training. Sizes (according to your height): up to 5'7", use 55 cm; 5'8" to 6', use 65 cm; 6' to 6'4", use 75 cm.

Dumbbells. To use while going through Levels B and C of Prong 1 to increase strength.

Ankle weights. Use throughout the entire rehab process to add resistance.

HYDRO-FIT INC.

160 Madison Street
Eugene, OR 97402-5031
Phone: 1-800-346-7295
Fax: 1-541-484-1443
Web: www.hydrofit.com

Sports therapy bar. Used for flotation and some water exercises.

Wave belt. Used as a flotation belt for water exercise program and to increase resistance when placed on ankles.

DJO/AIRCAST

790 Colombia Road
Plainfield, IN 46168
Phone: 1-800-526-8785
Fax: 1-800-457-4221
Web: www.betterbraces.com
E-mail: aircastorders@djortho.com

Knee Cryo/Cuff Autochill System. Allows you to have continual cold and compression while icing.

MY HEALTH AND SAFETY SUPPLY CO.

8003 Castleway Drive, Suite 200
Indianapolis, IN 46250
Phone: 1-888-462-6947
Fax: 1-317-524-1720
E-mail: My-SupportStockings.com

T.E.D. stockings. Thigh-high compression stockings are used postoperatively to reduce swelling and the risk of blood clots.

YAKTRAX

9221 Globe Center Drive
Morrisville, NC 27560
Phone: 1-800-446-7587
Fax: 1-919-314-1960
Web: www.yaktrax.com
E-mail: help@4implus.com

Yaktrax Walker, Yaktrax Pro. These items are great for those living around ice and snow. They slide right onto your shoes or boots and allow for slip-free outdoor exercise.

CWI MEDICAL

200 Allen Boulevard
Farmingdale, NY 11735
Phone: 1-866-588-3888
Fax: 1-866-588-3337
Web: www.cwimedical.com
E-mail: info@cwimedical.com

5-Prong Ice Grip Cane/Crutch Attachment (crampon). A crampon that can be easily attached to a cane or crutch during slippery conditions.

CYCLING EQUIPMENT AND OTHER FUN EXERCISE STUFF

You can use a stationary bike throughout your rehab program and life. There are many styles and brands, but the key is to get one that fits. Most indoor bikes can be adjusted to a fit similar to your outdoor bike (this is why you keep a measuring tape in your gym bag when traveling!). If a bike isn't comfortable, chances are you won't use it. Best bet: Set up your properly fit outdoor bike on an indoor trainer. Contact one of the following shops or Google "stationary bikes" for a dealer near you.

LITTLETON BIKE AND FITNESS

28 Cottage Street
Littleton, NH 03561
Phone: 603-444-3437
Fax: 603-444-6172
Web: www.littletonbike.com

Offers a full array of bikes and indoor exercise equipment plus expert bike fitting.

RHINO BIKE WORKS

1 Forster Street
Plymouth, NH 03264
Phone: 603-536-3919
Web: www.rhinobikeworks.com

Rhino sells road and mountain bicycles along with great cross-country ski equipment and other outdoor athletic gear.

S & W SPORTS

238 Main Street
Concord, NH 03301
Phone: 603-228-1441
Web: www.swsports.net

Wide variety of sports equipment suitable for rehabilitation and/or more advanced activities for each season of the year.

EDUCATIONAL RESOURCES

Trustworthy Web sites for further information about

- understanding even more about the knee, knee surgery, and sport psychology
- eating healthfully
- fitness and lifetime sports
- losing weight and keeping it off
- designing a personal routine to suit your individual needs and goals

Knee Surgery and Sport Psychology

Visit my Alpine Clinic Web site for helpful tips and additional information regarding your knee rehabilitation: www .THEALPINECLINIC.com. For more sport psychology—related questions, visit my Coaching Mental Excellence Web site at www.CMExcellence.com.

Total Knee Replacement

The American Association of Orthopaedic Surgeons (of which I am a member) offers free information about arthritis, osteoarthritis, total joint replacement, and medical terminology relating to knee surgery. The Web site is www .AAOS.org, or click on their Patient Information Center at http://orthoinfo.aaos.org/.

Orthopedic Sports Medicine

The American Orthopaedic Society for Sports Medicine (of which I am also a member) features an online library where you can research terms and conditions (using their search engine), at www.sportsmed.org/sml/edlit.asp. Their general Web address is www.sportsmed.org.

General Sports Medicine

To find a sports medicine doctor who is not a surgeon, see the American Medical Society of Sports Medicine's site at www.amssm.org. This organization offers a downloadable PDF document at http://amssm.org/Whatis.pdf., which details the qualifications and benefits of a sports medicine physician. You do not have to be an athlete to see or benefit from a sports medicine doctor!

Sport Psychology

In addition to www.CMExcellence.com, there is some good information at the Association for the Advancement of Applied Sport Psychology, www.aaasponline.org.

Training

The National Athletic Trainers' Association (NATA) Web site can be found at www.nata.org.

Personal Trainers

Personal trainers are a wonderful luxury, similar to a professional massage, that everyone should avail themselves of during an active life. I recommend a personal trainer at any point in the rehab process but especially once you get to Level C exercises and are adding in the aerobic training programs. Trainers help evaluate your form, give you important pointers, and make sure you are working smart, not necessarily just "hard." My one caveat is to make sure they familiarize themselves with my rehab program and don't just treat you like any other client. Multiple sessions in that first year post-op are great and everyone, bad knees or not, should have a personal training session annually to celebrate their birthday!

To find a trainer near you:

- Ask your friends and coworkers.
- Ask your doctors.
- Ask your doctors' nurses (nurses know everything).
- If you belong to a health club, ask about the trainers on staff or in the area.
- Go to your local bookstore or library and browse through books by trainers. If you like what the trainer says, check the author bio to see if he or she lives near you.

FITNESS AND NUTRITION

One of the most comprehensive sources for information is the U.S. Department of Health and Human Services, which offers information on everything from medications to surgery, up-to-date info on weight loss, fitness, and healthy lifestyles. Go to www.hhs.gov or write to HHS, 200 Independence Avenue, SW, Washington, DC 20201 for more information.

The President's Council on Physical Fitness and Sports's Web site, www.fitness.gov, is very useful.

The Centers for Disease Control at www.cdc.gov offer a wealth of helpful information including guidelines and tips on fitness. "Physical Fitness for Everyone" is their focus in this link: www.cdc.gov/nccdphp/dnpa/physical/components.

A very helpful Web site is www.healthierus.gov/nutrition .html. The American Dietetic Association offers a valuable resource as well, at www.eatright.org.

GLOSSARY

Aerobic. Literally, "with oxygen." Usually refers to workouts you can do for a long time (e.g., cycling or jogging).

Allograft. Using tendons from a cadaver to help repair ACL injuries.

Anaerobic. Literally, "without oxygen." Short bursts of activity such as weight lifting or sprinting that your body can sustain for only seconds (as opposed to many minutes, as in aerobic activities).

Anesthesia. Loss or removing of the sensation of pain.

Anterior cruciate ligament (ACL). One of the "crossing" (cruciate) ligaments in the center of your knee, connecting the femur to the tibia.

Anti-inflammatory medicines. Drugs like aspirin, Motrin, naprosyn, and Aleve that often make your knee feel better by reducing swelling and inflammation. All run the risk of upsetting the stomach and possibly ulcers with long-term use.

Arthritis. *Arth* means "joint" and *itis* means "inflammation." Most knee arthritis is not actually inflammatory but wear and tear to the surface cartilage (arthrosis). You say "arthritis" and I say "arthrosis," but both result in pain and stiffness.

Arthroscope. A lighted tube with a videocamera on one end, used for arthroscopic surgery.

Arthroscopy/arthroscopic surgery. An arthroscope is inserted into a joint ("arth"). More holes are made into the joint for instruments to perform the surgery.

Articular (surface) cartilage. Cartilage that caps the end of your bones; it starts out smooth but gets worn and crunchy with age or injury.

Autograft. Using tendons from elsewhere in the body to help reconstruct an ACL.

Background noise. Things in your life that distract you from the important stuff.

Cartilage. The cushioning structures in your knee made up of collagen fibers; the two basic types are articular and meniscal.

Co-contraction. Contracting two opposing muscles at the same time, such as quads and hamstrings.

Collateral ligament. A ligament on the side of a joint, e.g., medial collateral ligament of the knee.

Concentric. In exercise-speak, describes lifting a weight by contracting (shortening) a muscle.

Core. The muscles of your abdomen, back, hips, and shoulders. Without strength and stability here, legs and arms work harder and are more prone to injury.

Crampons. Spikes you can buy to put on the bottom of your crutches (or shoes) to keep from slipping on ice and snow (see Resources).

Cross-training. Using multiple sports and activities to maintain fitness while avoiding boredom and overuse injuries. Folks in places with seasonal changes do this naturally. Those in warmer climates must be more careful to vary their workout routines.

Deliberate practice. Performing a movement with concentration and attention to precision, preferably with coaching.

Eccentric. In weight rooms and exercise class, it describes lowering a weight so your muscles are working against gravity (a great way to strengthen muscles).

End-stage arthritis. Sometimes called "bone-on-bone" arthritis. This means the knee really hurts and it's time for a TKR.

Extension. Straightening the knee.

Flexion. Bending the knee.

Gait. Your walking pattern.

Gluteals/gluteus maximus, medius, minimus. Your hip (buttock) muscles.

Hamstrings. The muscles on the back of your thighs.

Hip. Ball-and-socket joint between your pelvis bone and the top of your femur (thighbone).

Hyperextension. Extending the knee past straight or "zero degrees" (aka "back knee").

Inflammation. The body's response to injury—swelling, pain, redness, heat, and limitation of motion.

Isophysiology. Exercises that make sense to your body by allowing full motion and continual resistance. Best example is water exercise.

IV. Intravenous line that allows fluids and medicine to be placed directly into your veins.

Joint. Where two bones come together.

Ligament. A ropelike structure connecting bone to bone, e.g., medial collateral ligament, anterior cruciate ligament, and posterior cruciate ligament.

Magnetic resonance image (MRI). A sophisticated radiological study that shows "soft tissues" (ligaments, cartilage, tendons) as well as bone. X-rays show only the bones and other calcified tissues.

Medial collateral ligament (MCL). The most frequently injured knee ligament, on the inner side of the knee. It usually heals without surgery.

Meniscal cartilage/meniscus. Pieces of gristle that live between your femur and tibia. They serve as cushions and stabilizers.

Meniscal repair. Putting stitches in the meniscus as opposed to removing the torn bits.

Microfracture/multiple drilling: Making holes in the end of your bone to stimulate healing of articular (surface) cartilage.

Mosaicplasty. Procedure that takes cartilage from a healthy part of the knee to repair surface cartilage damage.

Movement patterns. The motions that your body performs daily in both work and sport that lead to muscle memory. This memory can be lost if not practiced, such as before and after surgery.

Muscle. Multiple fibers that contract and extend to provide movement.

Musculoskeletal system. Consists of muscles and bones.

Passive. Letting someone or something else do the work, e.g., a therapist, machine, or gravity.

Posterior cruciate ligament (PCL). Less frequently injured ligament located behind the ACL.

Quadriceps/quads. The muscles on the front of the thighs that straighten the knee.

Reps. Repetitions of an exercise.

Resistive exercise. Exercise where your body works against resistance, most often weights, water exercise, or some type of rubber bands, cords, etc.

RICE. Acronym for rest, ice, compression, and elevation.

Sets. A group of exercise reps.

Soft workout. Anything that doesn't pound on your knee. Water is the ultimate soft workout, followed by cycling.

Elliptical machines are going away from soft, and running is definitely not soft.

Spinal anesthetic. Medicine placed through a thin needle into your back that numbs your body from the waist down.

Sutures. The materials surgeons use to close a wound. They come out of the knee anywhere from five to fourteen days after surgery, depending on surgeon's preference, length of the wound, etc. Also called stitches, staples.

T.E.D. stockings. White, thigh-high stockings that hold your bandages in place, keep the swelling down, and help guard against blood clots.

Tendon. A ropelike structure connecting muscle to bone.

Total knee replacement (TKR). Resurfacing of the articular (surface) cartilage at the end of the knee bone (femur, tibia, and patella) with a combination of metal and plastic components.

Training. The process of improving health and performance via a planned program of aerobic and anaerobic movements.

Viscosupplementation. The injection of a thick fluid into an arthritic knee to reduce pain and improve mobility.

X-rays. Pictures of your knee that show the bones but not the "soft tissues" (cartilage, ligaments).